Handbook of Nitro Sedation

Steven Goldenberg

Nitrous Oxide guide

Nitrous oxide is an unscented, dreary, non-combustible gas. While nitrous oxide isn't combustible, it will uphold burning in a similar way as oxygen. It prompts a condition of happiness, making sense of its epithet, 'giggling gas.' Nitrous oxide is the most un-powerful inhalational sedative. Contrasted with other sedative specialists, nitrous oxide causes insignificant impacts on breath and hemodynamics. It can't be a sole sedative specialist and is frequently joined with an additional intense and unpredictable sedative. The mix of pain relieving and sedative impacts makes nitrous oxide an important assistant. This action frames the signs, system of activity, strategies for organization, critical antagonistic impacts, contraindications, observing, and poisonousness of nitrous oxide, so suppliers can guide patient treatment to ideal results in sedation and different circumstances where nitrous oxide has helpful advantages.

Nitrous oxide is an unscented, drab, non-combustible gas. While nitrous oxide isn't combustible, it will uphold burning in a similar way as oxygen. It prompts a condition of happiness, making sense of its moniker, 'giggling gas.'

Nitrous oxide is the most un-intense inhalational sedative. Nitrous oxide requires a grouping of 104% to arrive at one least alveolar focus (Macintosh). Consequently it can't be a sole sedative specialist, and it is frequently joined with an additional intense and unpredictable sedative. The blend of pain relieving and sedative impacts makes nitrous oxide an important assistant. Nitrous oxide has a low blood solvency (blood-gas segment coefficient of 0.47), prompting a fast beginning and balanced. The low dissolvability prompts a concentrating impact for managed unstable specialists in the lungs and is known as the second gas effect.

Nitrous oxide can be utilized for general sedation, procedural sedation, dental sedation, and to treat serious agony. Nitrous oxide's powerful pain relieving properties can be helpful in giving absence of pain in settings like the obstetrical ward or crisis division. Its organization is much of the time a half combination of oxygen in these settings. Contrasted with other sedative specialists, nitrous oxide causes insignificant impacts on breath and hemodynamics. It prompts diminished flowing volume and expanded respiratory rate however limits generally minute ventilation. Nitrous oxide prompts direct myocardial wretchedness, however nitrous oxide's thoughtful excitement diminishes this impact, and the net impact is negligible. Not at all like other unstable sedatives, has nitrous oxide had no muscle unwinding properties.

Nitrous oxide is likewise being researched as an expected specialist for treatment-safe sadness. Be that as it may, further broad exploration is needed.

Instrument of Activity

Nitrous oxide has various supraspinal and spinal targets. The sedative impact of nitrous oxide is through non-serious NMDA hindrance in the focal sensory system. The pain relieving impacts happen by delivering endogenous narcotics that follow up on narcotic receptors; its pain relieving activities are like morphine. The anxiolytic impacts are through GABA-An initiation. Nitrous oxide has a focal thoughtful invigorating movement that supports circulatory strain, foundational vascular opposition, and cardiovascular result. Nitrous oxide animates cerebral blood stream and increments intracranial pressure.

Pharmacokinetics

Assimilation: Breathed in nitrous oxide is quickly consumed through alveoli. The beginning of activity is inside 2 to 5 mins.

Appropriation: Nitrous oxide might deliver the second-gas result on the grounds that nitrous oxide diffuses more quickly across alveolar cellular layers than different gases. The quick exit of nitrous oxide from the alveoli brings about leftover alveolar gases being concentrated, hence speeding up nitrous oxide take-up into the blood and speeding the beginning of sedation. Nitrous oxide has a Macintosh of 105%. Insignificant Alveolar Focus (Macintosh) connects with the power of unpredictable sedative specialists. It is characterized as the base alveolar convergence of breathed in sedative at which half of individuals don't move in light of poisonous improvements. Consequently N2O is a feeble sedative inhalational specialist however makes great pain relieving impacts. The inversion might happen toward the finish of sedation when nitrous oxide enters the alveoli undeniably more quickly, causing oxygen weakening inside the alveoli and may cause dissemination hypoxia.

Digestion: Nitrous oxide (a follow sum) is used through decrease by anaerobic microscopic organisms in the stomach.

Organization

Nitrous oxide organization is through inward breath using a straightforward facial covering, laryngeal veil aviation route, or an endotracheal tube. Organization of nitrous oxide as per the European Culture of Anesthesiology Team on Nitrous Oxide is given below.

For general sedation, nitrous oxide (50 to 70%) is utilized. Be that as it may, because of its low power, it cannot be utilized as a solitary sedative specialist; consequently it is joined with different specialists. Uniquely assigned gear for overseeing NO should be utilized to discover centralizations of half NO and half oxygen. Conversely, with dental mechanical assembly, the gadget supported for obstetric use doesn't permit the clinician to change the extent of gases.

Acceptance: The blend of lower solubility's in blood and various tissues makes N2O quite possibly of the quickest sedative specialist. N2O take-up in the lungs further develops the blood centralizations of correspondingly managed other unstable inward breath specialists and oxygen, prompting quicker enlistment and worked on blood vessel oxygenation.

Support: N2O is blended in with various medications during upkeep on account of its deficient sedative power. As examined above, nitrous oxide has a Macintosh of 105%, yet the arrangement of adequate oxygen conveyance blocks the organization of fixations over 70-75%, hence restricting its utilization to 0.7 Macintosh. Consolidating propofol with nitrous oxide for dental sedation diminishes propofol prerequisites and decreases the hypotensive impacts contrasted with propofol alone.

Development: Nitrous oxide animates rising up out of sedation. Moreover, nitrous oxide has a short end half-time; thus waste of time from the mind is quick a result of its lower lipid solvency, prompting fast recovery.

Use in Unambiguous Patient Populaces

Patients with Renal Weakness: No data is given in the maker's naming to portion changes in patients with renal disability.

Patients with Hepatic Hindrance: No data is given in the producer's naming to portion changes in patients with hepatic weakness.

Pregnancy Contemplations: As indicated by ACOG (American School of Obstetricians and Gynecologists), rules half nitrous oxide with half oxygen is utilized during work and for post pregnancy perinea fix. It is critical to perceive that nitrous oxide crosses the placenta, and it is quickly wiped out by youngsters upon the initiation of relaxing. In any case, ACOG and the American Culture of Anesthesiologists note that because of the expanded gamble of sedation and maternal hypoxemic episodes, nitrous oxide ought not to be joined with foundational narcotics or tranquilizers, or hypnotics.

Breastfeeding Contemplations: The half-existence of nitrous oxide in the mother is short, and the nitrous oxide isn't expected to be consumed by the baby. In this way, whenever utilized as a component of general sedation, breastfeeding can be begun after the mother has recuperated enough from anesthesia.

Unfriendly Impacts

Unfriendly impacts of nitrous include:

Respiratory Gloom: When utilized alone, nitrous makes restricted respiratory impacts, yet when utilized in mix with different narcotics, hypnotics, or narcotics, it can potentiate the respiratory depressant impacts of these specialists.

Dispersion hypoxia: Following stopping of nitrous oxide, the focus angle between the gases in the lung and alveolar dissemination quickly turns around, prompting fast oxygen weakening in the alveoli and resulting hypoxia, and 100 percent oxygen organization ought to follow nitrous oxide discontinuance.

Postoperative Queasiness and Spewing: Nitrous has an expanded gamble of postoperative sickness and retching (PONV) contrasted and different specialists, however this is controllable with prophylactic enemy of emetics. The Conundrum I preliminary showed an expanded occurrence of PONV with nitrous oxide use. The Conundrum II preliminary showed that extreme PONV with nitrous oxide use is more normal in methodology enduring north of 2 hours. This concentrate additionally showed nitrous oxide isn't related with expanded mortality, cardiovascular intricacies, or wound infections.

Fever, aspiratory atelectasis, and irresistible difficulties

Hyperhomocysteinemia: Nitrous oxide irreversibly oxidizes the cobalt particle of vitamin b12 and lessens the movement of vitaminb12 subordinate chemicals, for example, methionine synthetizes which can likewise prompt megaloblastic anemia.

Sub-acute myeloneuropathy: Nitrous oxide use turmoil can cause an extreme yet possibly reversible myeloneuropathy described by axonal sensorimotor neuropathy.

Contraindications

Numerous contraindications to nitrous use are relative and may fluctuate in view of the supplier. These include:

Fundamentally sick patients: Nitrous oxide inactivates methionine synthase by means of oxidation of the cobalt in vitamin B12 and may prompt megaloblastic frailty. This protein is fundamental for vitamin B12 and folate digestion and assumes a part in DNA and RNA blend and the union of different substances. In any case sound patients, the effect is subclinical. Notwithstanding, this might prompt neurologic or hematologic outcomes in fundamentally sick patients and ought to be stayed away from.

Extreme cardiovascular infection: Methionine synthase is likewise expected to change over homocysteine to methionine, and raised serum homocysteine levels are related with an expanded gamble for unfavorable coronary occasions.

The clinician ought to try not to involve nitrous oxide in extreme cardiovascular illness, yet further examinations are expected to decide the real effect.

The main trimester of pregnancy: Because of the above-referred to effect on B12 and folate digestion, nitrous use isn't suggested in the primary trimester of pregnancy.

Pneumothorax, little entrails deterrent, center ear medical procedure, and retinal medical procedures make an intraocular gas bubble: Nitrous oxide is multiple times more solvent than nitrogen. Nitrous oxide diffuses more quickly into shut spaces than nitrogen can diffuse out, prompting expanded gas volume and strain inside shut spaces. Subsequently nitrous oxide is contraindicated in pneumothorax, little gut block, center ear medical procedure, and retinal medical procedures including the making of an intraocular gas bubble. In laparoscopic cases, nitrous oxide can amass in the pneumoperitoneum, and some stay away from its utilization.

Serious mental issues: Nitrous oxide can cause dreaming and mind flights and ought to be stayed away from in patients with serious mental issues.

Pneumonic hypertension: Nitrous oxide can increment pneumonic supply route and wedge pressures by means of thoughtful excitement, and clinicians frequently stay away from it in patients with aspiratory hypertension.

Head and neck techniques with searing use: While nitrous oxide is non-combustible, it upholds ignition, and its utilization ought to be kept away from in these procedures.

Debilitated cognizance

Observing

No particular observing is essential for nitrous oxide use. An in-line oxygen analyzer with a caution ought to be utilized to forestall the conveyance of a hypoxic gas combination. Present day sedative machines have safeguard components to forestall this (nitrous oxide-oxygen proportioning frameworks). Standard ASA observing is vital while overseeing nitrous oxide for any indication.

The rooms where NO is used ought to be checked for appropriate ventilation, squander gas rummaging, and risk correspondence. Furthermore, a pin-file wellbeing framework ought to be observed to forestall the irregular connection of a nonoxygen tank to the oxygen portal.

As indicated by the American Culture of Anesthesiology, intermittent evaluation of aviation route patency, oxygen immersion, and respiratory rate ought to be finished during rise and recuperation, with specific thoughtfulness regarding checking oxygenation and ventilation. Hemodynamic boundaries ought to be observed during development and recovery.

Harmfulness

While nitrous oxide inactivates methionine synthase, intraoperative use brings about a transient metabolic irregularity that before long switches after supplanting the debasing compound.

At the point when nitrous oxide is utilized repetitively (during word related openness or as a medication of misuse), it might prompt megaloblastic sickliness with neurologic brokenness. This present circumstance likewise may happen in patients with a lack of unnoticed coalmine (veggie lovers, malignant paleness, genetic problems of coalman, and folate digestion). Sub-acute joined degeneration of the spinal line (SACD) and passing is accounted for with rehashed openness for a situation of an intriguing intrinsic methylenetetrahydrofolate reeducates (MTHFR) deficiency.

Improving Medical care Group Results

Nitrous oxide is a broadly involved choice for work absence of pain and dentistry. One justification behind restricted use in the US is the restricted accessibility of sedation inclusion. The nursing staff has shown that nitrous oxide organization and the board are protected, practical work absence of pain options. A meta-examination of 35 RCTs showed no distinctions in the in-clinic casualty paces of nitrous oxide-based and nitrous sans oxide sedation. In any case, clinicians ought to stay away from nitrous oxide in patients with poor pneumonic capability and patients at higher gamble for postoperative queasiness and vomiting. [Level 1] Confirmed enlisted nurture anesthetists(CRNAs) regulated nitrous oxide has likewise given procedural sedation in pediatric radiology, bringing about less unfriendly impacts and a faster re-visitation of benchmark than oral midazolam.

Hospitalists or internists normally check preoperative assessment. Anesthetists and CRNAs regulate nitrous oxide. The perioperative drug store group ought to aid prescription acquirement, advance safe medicine use as per guidelines, and survey preoperative and post anesthesia care unit (PACU) orders. At the point when utilized in obstetric settings, the protected and fitting utilization of nitrous oxide requires coordination and correspondence of an interprofessional group of obstetricians, primatologists, guaranteed enrolled nurture anesthetists (CRNAs), anesthesiologists, neonatal escalated care units, and biomedical and risk the board departments.

Nitrous oxide is likewise broadly utilized in dental settings. Dental hygienists and associates are approved to control nitrous oxide in specific states. As indicated by CDC, ongoing word related openness to nitrous oxide might prompt neurological inconveniences and an expanded gamble of premature delivery. Thus, an interprofessional approach between dental specialists, dental hygienists, and dental associates is required while directing nitrous oxide to forestall word related hazards.

A meta-examination of 35 RCTs showed no distinctions in the in-clinic casualty paces of nitrous oxide-based and nitrous without oxide sedation. In any case, clinicians ought to keep away from nitrous oxide in patients with poor pneumonic capability and patients at higher gamble for postoperative sickness and vomiting.

nitrous oxide (N2O), likewise called nitrogen monoxide, giggling gas, or nitrous, one of a few oxides of nitrogen, a lackluster gas with lovely, sweetish smell and taste, which when breathed in produces obliviousness to torment went before by gentle mania, in some cases chuckling. (Since inward breath of modest quantities gives a short euphoric impact and nitrous oxide isn't against the law to have, the substance has been utilized as a sporting medication.) Nitrous oxide was found by the English physicist Joseph Priestley in 1772; another English scientist, Humphrey Davy, later named it and showed its physiological impact. A chief utilization of nitrous oxide is as a sedative in careful tasks of brief term; delayed inward breath causes demise. The gas is likewise utilized as a force in food vapor sprayers. In car hustling, nitrous oxide is infused into a motor's air admission; the additional oxygen permits the motor to consume more fuel per stroke. It is ready by the activity of zinc on weaken nitric corrosive, by the activity of hydroxylamine hydrochloride ($NH_2OH \cdot HCl$) on sodium nitrite ($NaNO_2$), and, most generally, by the deterioration of ammonium nitrate (NH_4NO_3).

Nonmetal, in material science, a substance having a limited enactment energy (band hole) for electron conduction. This implies that nonmetals show low (encasings) to direct (semiconductors) mass electrical conductivities, which increment with expanding temperature, and are dependent upon dielectric breakdown at high voltages and temperatures. Like metals, nonmetals might happen in the strong, fluid, or vaporous state. Nonetheless, not at all like metals, nonmetals show many the two mechanical and optical properties, going from fragile to plastic and from straightforward to murky.

According to a substance perspective, nonmetals might be separated into two classes:1) covalent materials, which contain molecules having little sizes, high electronegativity's, low valence opening to electron proportions, and an articulated propensity to shape negative particles in synthetic responses and negative oxidation states in their mixtures; 2) ionic materials, which contain both little and huge molecules. Particles might be framed by adding electrons to (little, electronegative iotas) or by separating electrons from (enormous, electropositive) molecules. In ionic materials, nonmetals exist either as monatomic anions (e. g., F-in Nave) or as constituents of polyatomic anions (e.g., N and O in the NO3-'s in NaNO3). At the point when as basic essential substances, around 25 or 22% of the realized components structure nonmetals at typical temperatures and tensions, remembering every one of the components for the S-block of the occasional table and roughly 58% of those in the P-block.

Ozone depleting substance

Ozone depleting substance, any gas that has the property of retaining infrared radiation (net intensity energy) produced from Earth's surface and reradiating it back to Earth's surface, hence adding to the nursery impact. Carbon dioxide, methane, and water fume are the main ozone harming substances. (Less significantly, superficial ozone, nitrous oxides, and fluorinated gases likewise trap infrared radiation.) Ozone harming substances significantly affect the energy financial plan of the Earth framework regardless of making up just a small portion of every single climatic gas. Groupings of ozone depleting substances have fluctuated significantly during Earth's set of experiences, and these varieties have driven significant environment changes at an extensive variety of timescales. As a general rule, ozone depleting substance fixations have been especially high during warm periods and low during cold periods.

Various cycles impact ozone harming substance fixations. Some, like structural exercises, work at timescales of millions of years, while others, like vegetation, soil, wetland, and sea sources and sinks, work at timescales of hundreds to millennia. Human exercises — particularly non-renewable energy source ignition since the Modern Unrest — are answerable for consistent expansions in air groupings of different ozone depleting substances, particularly carbon dioxide, methane, ozone, and chlorofluorocarbons (CFCs).

The impact of every ozone harming substance on Earth's environment relies upon its synthetic nature and its general fixation in the climate. A few gases have a high limit with regards to retaining infrared radiation or happen in huge amounts, while others have significantly lower capacities with regards to retention or happen just in follow sums. Radioactive compelling, as characterized by the Intergovernmental Board on Environmental Change (IPCC), is a proportion of the impact a given ozone depleting substance or other climatic variable (like sun powered irradiance or albedo) has on how much brilliant energy impinging upon Earth's surface. To grasp the overall impact of every ozone harming substance, supposed compelling qualities (given in watts per square meter) determined for the time span among 1750 and the current day are given beneath.

Significant ozone depleting substances

Water fume

Water fume is the strongest ozone harming substance in Earth's climate, however its way of behaving is in a general sense not the same as that of the other ozone depleting substances. The essential job of water fume isn't as an immediate specialist of radioactive constraining yet rather as an environment criticism — that is, as a reaction inside the environment framework that impacts the framework's proceeded with action. This qualification emerges on the grounds that how much water fume in the environment can't, by and large, be straightforwardly adjusted by human way of behaving yet is rather set via air temperatures. The hotter the surface, the more prominent the dissipation pace of water from the surface. Subsequently, expanded vanishing prompts a more prominent centralization of water fume in the lower environment fit for engrossing infrared radiation and emanating it back to the surface.

Carbon dioxide

Carbon dioxide (CO2) is the main ozone harming substance. Regular wellsprings of barometrical CO2 incorporate outgassing from volcanoes, the burning and normal rot of natural matter, and breath by high-impact (oxygen-utilizing) creatures. By and large, by a bunch of physical, compound, or natural cycles, called "sinks," that will generally eliminate CO2 from the climate. Critical regular sinks incorporate earthly vegetation, which takes up CO2 during photosynthesis.

Various maritime cycles likewise go about as carbon sinks. One such cycle, the "solvency siphon," includes the plummet of surface seawater containing broke down CO2. Another cycle, the "natural siphon," includes the take-up of broken up CO2 by marine vegetation and phytoplankton (little, free-drifting, photosynthetic organic entities) living in the upper sea or by other marine creatures that utilization CO2 to assemble skeletons and different designs made of calcium carbonate (CaCO3). As these organic entities lapse and tumble to the sea floor, their carbon is moved descending and in the end covered at profundity. A drawn out balance between these regular sources and sinks prompts the foundation, or normal, level of CO2 in the environment.

Conversely, human exercises increment environmental CO2 levels basically through the consuming of petroleum derivatives (mainly oil and coal, and optionally flammable gas, for use in transportation, warming, and power creation) and through the development of concrete. Other anthropogenic sources incorporate the consuming of woodlands and the getting free from land. Anthropogenic outflows presently represent the yearly arrival of around 7 gigatons (7 billion tons) of carbon into the air. Anthropogenic discharges are equivalent to roughly 3% of the complete emanations of CO2 by regular sources, and this intensified carbon load from human exercises far surpasses the balancing limit of normal sinks (by maybe as much as 2-3 gig tons each year).

CO2 has subsequently collected in the climate at a typical pace of 1.4 parts per million (ppm) by volume each year somewhere in the range of 1959 and 2006 and generally 2.0 ppm each year somewhere in the range of 2006 and 2018. Generally speaking, this pace of collection has been direct (that is, uniform over the long haul). Nonetheless, certain flow sinks, like the seas, could become sources from here on out. This might prompt a circumstance in which the convergence of barometrical CO_2 works at an outstanding rate (that is, at a pace of increment that is likewise expanding over the long run).

The regular foundation level of carbon dioxide shifts on timescales of millions of years because of slow changes in outgassing through volcanic action. For instance, approximately quite a while back, during the Cretaceous Time frame, CO_2 fixations seem to have been a few times higher than today (maybe near 2,000 ppm). Throughout recent years, CO_2 fixations have fluctuated over a far more modest reach (between about 180 and 300 ppm) in relationship with similar Earth orbital impacts connected to the approaching and going of the ice times of the Pleistocene age. By the mid-21st hundred years, CO_2 levels came to 384 ppm, which is around 37% over the regular foundation level of approximately 280 ppm that existed toward the start of the Modern Unrest. Climatic CO_2 levels proceeded to increment, and by 2018 they had reached 410 ppm. As per ice center estimations, such levels are accepted to be the most noteworthy in something like 800,000 years and, as per different lines of proof, might be the most noteworthy in somewhere around 5,000,000 years.

Radioactive constraining brought about via carbon dioxide differs in an around logarithmic design with the centralization of that gas in the climate. The logarithmic relationship happens as the consequence of an immersion impact wherein it turns out to be progressively troublesome, as CO2 fixations increment, for extra CO2 particles to additional impact the "infrared window" (a specific thin band of frequencies in the infrared locale that isn't consumed by barometrical gases). The logarithmic relationship predicts that the surface warming potential will ascend by generally a similar sum for each multiplying of CO2 fixation. At current paces of petroleum product use, a multiplying of CO2 fixations over preindustrial levels is supposed to occur by the center of the 21st hundred years (when CO2 focuses are projected to reach 560 ppm). A multiplying of CO2 fixations would address an increment of approximately 4 watts for each square meter of radiative constraining. Given ordinary evaluations of "environment responsiveness" without a trace of balancing factors, this energy increment would prompt a warming of 2 to 5 °C (3.6 to 9 °F) over preindustrial times. The complete radiative compelling by anthropogenic CO_2 discharges starting from the start of the modern age is around 1.66 watts per square meter.

Methane

Methane (CH_4) is the second most significant ozone depleting substance. CH_4 is stronger than CO_2 on the grounds that the radiative constraining delivered per atom is more noteworthy. Likewise, the infrared window is less immersed in the scope of frequencies of radiation consumed by CH_4, so more particles might fill in the district. In any case, CH_4 exists in far lower focuses than CO_2 in the climate, and its fixations by volume in the air are by and large estimated in parts per billion (ppb) as opposed to ppm. CH_4 likewise has an extensively more limited home time in the climate than CO_2 (the home time for CH_4 is around 10 years, contrasted and many years for CO_2).

Normal wellsprings of methane incorporate tropical and northern wetlands, methane-oxidizing microorganisms that feed on natural material consumed by termites, volcanoes, drainage vents of the ocean bottom in areas rich with natural dregs, and methane hydrates caught along the mainland racks of the seas and in polar permafrost. The essential normal sink for methane is the actual air, as methane responds promptly with the hydroxyl extremist (OH−) inside the lower atmosphere to frame CO_2 and water fume (H_2O). At the point when CH_4 arrives at the stratosphere, it is obliterated. Another normal sink is soil, where methane is oxidized by microscopic organisms.

Likewise with CO_2, human movement is expanding the CH_4 fixation quicker than it tends to be balanced by regular sinks. Anthropogenic sources right now represent roughly 70% of absolute yearly discharges, prompting significant expansions in fixation after some time. The major anthropogenic wellsprings of air CH_4 are rice development, domesticated animals cultivating, the consuming of coal and flammable gas, the burning of biomass, and the deterioration of natural matter in landfills. Future patterns are especially hard to expect. This is to a limited extent because of an inadequate comprehension of the environment inputs related with CH4 emanations. What's more, as human populaces develop, it is challenging to anticipate how potential changes in domesticated animals raising, rice development, and energy use will impact CH4 discharges.

It is accepted that an unexpected expansion in the grouping of methane in the air was liable for a warming occasion that raised typical worldwide temperatures by 4-8 °C (7.2-14.4 °F) more than two or three thousand years during the purported Paleocene-Eocene Warm Greatest (PETM). This episode occurred around quite a while back, and the ascent in CH4 seems to have been connected with a gigantic volcanic ejection that collaborated with methane-containing flood stores. Thus, a lot of vaporous CH4 were infused into the climate. It is challenging to know definitively how high these fixations were or the way in which long they persevered. At extremely high focuses, home seasons of CH4 in the climate can turn out to be a lot more noteworthy than the ostensible 10-year home time that applies today. By the by, almost certainly, these fixations arrived at a few ppm during the PETM.

Methane focuses likewise changed over a more modest reach (between approximately 350 and 800 ppb) in relationship with the Pleistocene ice age cycles. Preindustrial levels of CH4 in the environment were around 700 ppb, though levels surpassed 1,867 ppb in late 2018. (These fixations are well over the regular levels noticed for basically the beyond 650,000 years.) The net radiative compelling by anthropogenic CH4 outflows is around 0.5 watt per square meter — or about 33% the radiative constraining of CO2.

Lesser ozone harming substances

Superficial ozone

The following most critical ozone harming substance is surface, or low-level, ozone (O3). Surface O3 is a consequence of air contamination; it should be recognized from normally happening stratospheric O3, which plays a totally different part in the planetary radiation balance. The essential normal wellspring of surface O3 is the subsidence of stratospheric O3 from the upper environment. Interestingly, the essential anthropogenic wellspring of surface O3 is photochemical responses including the barometrical toxin carbon monoxide (CO). The best gauges of the regular centralization of surface O3 are 10 ppb, and the net radiative driving because of anthropogenic outflows of surface O3 is around 0.35 watt per square meter. Ozone focuses can ascend to unfortunate levels (that is, conditions where fixations meet or surpass 70 ppb for eight hours or longer) in urban areas inclined to photochemical exhaust cloud.

Nitrous oxides and fluorinated gases

Extra follow gases created by modern action that have nursery properties incorporate nitrous oxide (N2O) and fluorinated gases (halocarbons), the last option including CFCs, sulfur hexafluoride, hydro fluorocarbons (HFCs), and per fluorocarbons (PFCs). Nitrous oxide is liable for 0.16 watt per square meter radiative driving, while fluorinated gases are altogether answerable for 0.34 watt per square meter. Nitrous oxides have little foundation fixations because of normal natural responses in soil and water, though the fluorinated gases owe their reality essentially to modern sources.

Oxygen

Oxygen (O), nonmetallic substance component of Gathering 16 (Through, or the oxygen bunch) of the intermittent table. Oxygen is a dry, scentless, dull gas fundamental for living creatures, being taken up by creatures, which convert it to carbon dioxide; plants, thus, use carbon dioxide as a wellspring of carbon and return the oxygen to the environment. Oxygen structures compounds by response with basically some other component, as well as by responses that dislodge components from their blends with one another; as a rule, these cycles are joined by the development of intensity and light and in such cases are called ignitions. Its most significant compound is water.

Oxygen was found around 1772 by a Swedish physicist, Carl Wilhelm Scheele, who got it by warming potassium nitrate, mercuric oxide, and numerous different substances. An English scientist, Joseph Priestley, autonomously found oxygen in 1774 by the warm decay of mercuric oxide and distributed his discoveries that very year, three years before Scheele distributed. In 1775-80, French physicist Antoine-Laurent Lavoisier, with wonderful understanding, deciphered the job of oxygen in breath as well as ignition, disposing of the phlogiston hypothesis, which had been acknowledged up to that time; he noticed its inclination to frame acids by joining with a wide range of substances and likewise named the component oxygen (oxygène) from the Greek words for "corrosive previous."

Event and properties

At 46% of the mass, oxygen is the most ample component in Earth's outside layer. The extent of oxygen by volume in the air is 21% and by weight in seawater is 89%. In rocks, it is joined with metals and nonmetals as oxides that are acidic (like those of sulfur, carbon, aluminum, and phosphorus) or essential (like those of calcium, magnesium, and iron) and as saltlike mixtures that might be viewed as framed from the acidic and fundamental oxides, as sulfates, carbonates, silicates, aluminates, and phosphates. Abundant as they are, these strong mixtures are not valuable as wellsprings of oxygen, since partition of the component from its tight blends with the metal iotas is excessively costly.

Underneath −183 °C (−297 °F), oxygen is a light blue fluid; it becomes strong at about −218 °C (−361 °F). Unadulterated oxygen is 1.1 times heavier than air.

During breath, creatures and a few microbes take oxygen from the air and return to it carbon dioxide, though by photosynthesis, green plants acclimatize carbon dioxide within the sight of daylight and develop free oxygen. Practically all the free oxygen in the air is because of photosynthesis. Around 3 pieces of oxygen by volume disintegrate in 100 pieces of new water at 20 °C (68 °F), somewhat less in seawater. Disintegrated oxygen is fundamental for the breath of fish and other marine life.

Regular oxygen is a combination of three stable isotopes: oxygen-16 (99.759 percent), oxygen-17 (0.037 percent), and oxygen-18 (0.204 percent). A few misleadingly pre-arranged radioactive isotopes are known. The longest-lived, oxygen-15 (124-final part life), has been utilized to concentrate on breath in warm blooded animals.

Allotropy

Oxygen has two allotropic structures, diatomic (O2) and triatomic (O3, ozone). The properties of the diatomic structure propose that six electrons bond the particles and two electrons stay unpaired, representing the paramagnetic of oxygen. The three particles in the ozone particle don't lie along a straight line.

Ozone might be delivered from oxygen as per the condition:

The interaction, as composed, is endothermic (energy should be given to make it continue); change of ozone back into diatomic oxygen is advanced by the presence of progress metals or their oxides. Unadulterated oxygen is part of the way changed into ozone by a quiet electrical release; the response is additionally achieved by ingestion of bright light of frequencies around 250 nanometers (nm, the nanometre, equivalent to 10−9 meter); event of this cycle in the upper climate eliminates radiation that would be destructive to life on the outer layer of the Earth. The impactful smell of ozone is observable in bound regions in which there is starting of electrical gear, as in generator rooms. Ozone is light blue; its thickness is 1.658 times that of air, and it has a limit of −112 °C (−170 °F) at barometrical tension.

Ozone is a strong oxidizing specialist, equipped for switching sulfur dioxide over completely to sulfur trioxide, sulfides to sulfates, iodides to iodine (giving an insightful strategy to its assessment), and numerous natural mixtures to oxygenated subordinates like aldehydes and acids. The transformation by ozone of hydrocarbons from auto fumes gases to these acids and aldehydes adds to the bothering idea of exhaust cloud. Monetarily, ozone has been utilized as a substance reagent, as a sanitizer, in sewage treatment, water refinement, and fading materials.

Preparative strategies

Creation strategies picked for oxygen rely on the amount of the component wanted. Lab systems incorporate the accompanying:

1. Warm decay of specific salts, for example, potassium chlorate or potassium nitrate:

The decay of potassium chlorate is catalyzed by oxides of change metals; manganese dioxide (pyrolusite, MnO_2) is oftentimes utilized. The temperature important to impact the advancement of oxygen is decreased from 400 °C to 250 °C by the impetus.

2. Warm disintegration of oxides of weighty metals:

Scheele and Priestley utilized mercury (II) oxide in their arrangements of oxygen.

3. Warm disintegration of metal peroxides or of hydrogen peroxide:

An early business methodology for separating oxygen from the climate or for production of hydrogen peroxide relied upon the arrangement of barium peroxide from the oxide as displayed in the situations.

4. Electrolysis of water containing little extents of salts or acids to permit conduction of the electric flow:

Business creation and use

At the point when expected in weight amounts, oxygen is ready by the fragmentary refining of fluid air. Of the primary parts of air, oxygen has the most elevated edge of boiling over and thusly is less unpredictable than nitrogen and argon. The interaction exploits the way that when a compacted gas is permitted to extend, it cools. Significant stages in the activity incorporate the accompanying: (1) Air is sifted to eliminate particulates; (2) dampness and carbon dioxide are taken out by assimilation in antacid; (3) the air is packed and the intensity of pressure eliminated by normal cooling techniques; (4) the compacted and cooled air is passed into curls contained in a chamber; (5) a part of the compacted air (at around 200 environments pressure) is permitted to extend in the chamber, cooling the loops; (6) the extended gas is gotten back to the blower with different ensuing development and pressure steps coming about at last in liquefaction of the packed air at a temperature of −196 °C; (7) the fluid air is permitted to warm to distil first the light uncommon gases, then, at that point, the nitrogen, leaving fluid oxygen. Different fractionations will create an item sufficiently unadulterated (99.5 percent) for most modern purposes.

The steel business is the biggest customer of unadulterated oxygen in "blowing" high carbon steel — that is, volatilizing carbon dioxide and other nonmetal contaminations in a faster and more handily controlled process than if air were utilized. The treatment of sewage by oxygen holds guarantee for more proficient treatment of fluid effluents than other synthetic cycles. Burning of squanders in shut frameworks utilizing unadulterated oxygen has become significant. The alleged LOX of rocket oxidizer powers is fluid oxygen; the utilization of LOX relies on the action of room programs. Unadulterated oxygen is utilized in submarines and jumping chimes.

Business oxygen or oxygen-advanced air has supplanted standard air in the compound business for the production of such oxidation-controlled synthetic substances as acetylene, ethylene oxide, and methanol. Clinical utilizations of oxygen remember use for oxygen tents, inhalators, and pediatric hatcheries. Oxygen-enhanced vaporous sedatives guarantee life support during general sedation. Oxygen is critical in various ventures that utilization ovens.

Synthetic properties and responses

The enormous upsides of the electronegativity and the electron liking of oxygen are ordinary of components that show just nonmetallic way of behaving. All in its mixtures, oxygen expects a negative oxidation state which would be considered normal from the two half-filled external orbitals. When these orbitals are filled by electron move, the oxide particle O^{2-} is made. In peroxides (species containing the particle O_2^{2-}) it is expected that every oxygen has a charge of -1. This property of tolerating electrons by complete or halfway exchange characterizes an oxidizing specialist. At the point when such a specialist responds with an electron-giving substance, its own oxidation state is brought down. The change (bringing down), from the zero to the −2 state on account of oxygen, is known as a decrease. Oxygen might be considered the "first" oxidizing specialist, the terminology used to depict oxidation and decrease being founded on this conduct common of oxygen.

As depicted in the part on allotropy, oxygen shapes the diatomic species, O2, under typical circumstances and, also, the triatomic species ozone, O3. There is some proof for an entirely shaky tetratomic animal groups, O4. In the sub-atomic diatomic structure there are two unpaired electrons that lie in anticoding orbitals. The paramagnetic way of behaving of oxygen affirms the presence of such electrons.

The extreme reactivity of ozone is once in a while made sense of by proposing that one of the three oxygen particles is in a "nuclear" state; on responding, this iota is separated from the O3 particle, leaving sub-atomic oxygen.

The sub-atomic species, O2, isn't particularly receptive at typical (surrounding) temperatures and tensions. The nuclear species, O, is undeniably more receptive. The energy of separation (O2 → 2O) is huge at 117.2 kilocalories per mole.

Oxygen has an oxidation condition of −2 in a large portion of its mixtures. It frames an enormous scope of covalently reinforced compounds, among which are oxides of nonmetals, like water (H_2O), sulfur dioxide (SO_2), and carbon dioxide (CO_2); natural mixtures like alcohols, aldehydes, and carboxylic acids; normal acids, for example, sulfuric (H_2SO_4), carbonic (H_2CO_3), and nitric (HNO_3); furthermore, relating salts, for example, sodium sulfate (Na_2SO_4), sodium carbonate (Na_2CO_3), and sodium nitrate ($NaNO_3$). Oxygen is available as the oxide particle, O^{2-}, in the translucent design of strong metallic oxides like calcium oxide, CaO. Metallic superoxide's, like potassium superoxide, KO_2, contain the O_2^- particle, though metallic peroxides, for example, barium peroxide, BaO_2, contain the O_2^{2-} particle.

Sir Humphrey Davy

Sir Humphrey Davy, in full Sir Humphrey Davy, Baronet, (conceived December 17, 1778, Penance, Cornwall, Britain — kicked the bucket May 29, 1829, Geneva, Switzerland), English physicist who found a few synthetic components (counting sodium and potassium) and mixtures, developed the digger's security light, and became one of the best types of the logical technique.

Early life

Davy was the senior child of working class guardians who claimed a home in Ludgvan, Cornwall, Britain. He was taught at the language structure school in adjacent Penzance and, in 1793, at Truro. In 1795, a year after the demise of his dad, Robert, he was apprenticed to a specialist and pharmacist, and he trusted in the long run to qualify in medication. A rich, warm, and famous chap, of speedy mind and exuberant creative mind, he was attached to forming refrains, drawing, making firecrackers, fishing, shooting, and gathering minerals. He wanted to meander, one pocket loaded up with fishing supplies and the other with rock examples; he never lost his serious love of nature and, especially, of mountain and water view.

While still a young, candid and to some degree reckless, Davy had plans for a volume of sonnets, however he started the serious investigation of science in 1797, and these dreams "escaped before the voice of truth." He was become a close acquaintence with by Davies Jubilant (later Gilbert; leader of the Illustrious Society, 1827-30), who offered him the utilization of his library in Tradea and took him to a science research facility that was exceptional for that day. There he shaped firmly free perspectives on subjects existing apart from everything else, like the idea of intensity, light, and power and the compound and actual teachings of Antoine Lavoisier. On Gilbert's proposal, he was selected (1798) substance director of the Pneumatic Foundation, established at Clifton to ask into the conceivable remedial purposes of different gases. Davy chased down the issue with trademark energy, manifesting a remarkable ability for trial request. In his little confidential lab, he arranged and breathed in nitrous oxide (chuckling gas) to test a case that it was the "guideline of virus," that is, caused illnesses. He researched the organization of the oxides and acids of nitrogen, as well as alkali, and convinced his logical and scholarly companions, including Samuel Taylor Coleridge, Robert Southey, and Peter Imprint Roget, to report the impacts of breathing in nitrous oxide. He almost lost his own life breathing in water gas, a combination of hydrogen and carbon monoxide some of the time utilized as fuel.

The record of his work, distributed as Explores, Synthetic and Philosophical, Essentially Concerning Nitrous Oxide, or Dephlogisticated Nitrous Air, and Its Breath (1800), quickly settled Davy's standing, and he was welcome to address at the recently established Illustrious Foundation of Extraordinary England in London, where he moved in 1801, with the commitment of help from the English American researcher Sir Benjamin Thompson (Count von Rumford), the English naturalist Sir Joseph Banks, and the English scientific expert and physicist Henry Cavendish in advancing his investigates — e.g., on voltaic cells, early types of electric batteries. His painstakingly ready and practiced addresses quickly became significant social capabilities and added enormously to the notoriety of science and the establishment. In 1802 he became teacher of science. His obligations incorporated an exceptional investigation of tanning: he tracked down catechu, the concentrate of a tropical plant, as successful as and less expensive than the typical oak concentrates, and his distributed record was for some time utilized as a leather expert's aide. In 1803 he was conceded an individual of the Imperial Society and a privileged individual from the Dublin Society and conveyed the first of a yearly series of talks before the leading body of farming. This prompted his Components of Horticultural Science (1813), the main efficient turn out accessible for a long time. For his explores on voltaic cells, tanning, and mineral examination, he got the Copley Decoration in 1805. He was chosen secretary of the Regal Society in 1807.

Significant revelations

Davy early reasoned that the development of power in basic electrolytic cells came about because of compound activity and that synthetic blend happened between substances of inverse charge. He thusly contemplated that electrolysis, the communications of electric flows with synthetic mixtures, offered the most probable method for disintegrating all substances to their components. These perspectives were made sense of in 1806 in his talk "On A few Synthetic Organizations of Power," for which, notwithstanding the way that Britain and France were at war, he got the Napoleon Prize from the Institut de France

(1807). This work drove straightforwardly to the disconnection of sodium and potassium from their mixtures (1807) and of the basic earth metals magnesium, calcium, strontium, and barium from their mixtures (1808). He additionally found boron (by warming borax with potassium), hydrogen telluride, and hydrogen phosphide (phosphine). He showed the right connection of chlorine to hydrochloric corrosive and the indefensibility of the previous name (oxymuriatic corrosive) for chlorine; this refuted Lavoisier's hypothesis that all acids contained oxygen. He likewise showed that chlorine is a compound component, and examinations intended to uncover oxygen in chlorine fizzled. He made sense of the dying activity of chlorine (through its freedom of oxygen from water) and found two of its oxides (1811 and 1815), yet his perspectives on the idea of chlorine were questioned.

In 1810 and 1811 he addressed to huge crowds at Dublin (on rural science, the components of substance reasoning, geography) and got £1,275 in charges, as well as the privileged level of LL.D., from Trinity School. In 1812 he was knighted by the Ruler Official (April 8), conveyed a goodbye talk to individuals from the Imperial

Establishment (April 9), and wedded Jane Apreece, a rich widow notable in friendly and scholarly circles in Britain and Scotland (April 11). He likewise distributed the initial segment of the Components of Synthetic Way of thinking, which contained his very own lot work. His arrangement was excessively aggressive, in any case, and nothing further showed up. Its finish, as indicated by Swedish physicist Jöns Jacob Berzelius, would have "high level the study of science an entire 100 years."

His last significant demonstration at the Imperial Organization, of which he stayed privileged teacher, was to talk with the youthful Michael Faraday, later to become one of Britain's extraordinary researchers, who became lab partner there in 1813 and went with the Davys on a European visit (1813-15). By consent of Napoleon, he went through France, meeting numerous conspicuous researchers, and was introduced to the sovereign Marie Louise. With the guide of a little convenient research facility and of different establishments in France and Italy, he explored the substance "X" (later called iodine), whose properties and closeness to chlorine he immediately found; further work on different mixtures of iodine and chlorine was finished before he arrived at Rome. He likewise dissected numerous examples of old style colors and demonstrated that precious stone is a type of carbon.

Later long periods of Sir Humphrey Davy

Soon after his return, he examined, for the General public for Forestalling Mishaps in Coal Mineshafts, the circumstances under which combinations of firedamp and air detonate. This prompted the creation of the excavator's security light and to resulting investigates on fire, for which he got the Rumford decorations (gold and silver) from the Imperial Society and, from the northern mine proprietors, a help of plate (in the end offered to establish the Davy Decoration). Subsequent to being made a baronet in 1818, he again went to Italy, asking into volcanic activity and trying and, sadly, failing to track down an approach to unrolling the papyri found at Herculaneum. In 1820 he became leader of the Imperial Society, a position he held until 1827. In 1823-25 he was related with the lawmaker and essayist John Wilson Croker in establishing the Athenaeum Club, of which he was a unique legal administrator, and with the pioneer lead representative Sir Stamford Wagers in establishing the Zoological Society and in assisting the plan for zoological nurseries in Official's Park, London (opened in 1828). During this period, he inspected attractive peculiarities brought about by power and electrochemical techniques for forestalling saltwater consumption of copper sheathing on ships through iron and zinc plates. However the defensive standards were clarified, impressive fouling happened, and the technique's disappointment enormously vexed him. Be that as it may, he was, as he expressed, "wore out." His Bakerian address for 1826, "On the Connection of Electrical and Substance Changes," contained his latest contemplations on electrochemistry and procured him the Illustrious Society's Regal Decoration.

Davy's wellbeing was by then bombing quickly; in 1827 he left for Europe and, in the late spring, had to leave the administration of the Imperial Society, being prevailed by Davies Gilbert. Swearing off business and field sports, Davy composed Salmonia: or on the other hand long stretches of Fly Fishing (1828), a book on fishing (after the way of Isaak Walton) that contained etchings from his own drawings. After a last, short visit to Britain, he got back to Italy, settling at Rome in February 1829 — "a ruin among ruins." However halfway deadened through stroke, he went through his last month's composing a progression of discoursed, distributed post mortem as Encouragements in Movement, or the Last Days of a Logician (1830).

Joseph Priestley

Joseph Priestley, (conceived Walk 13, 1733, Bristol Field head, close to Leeds, Yorkshire [now West Yorkshire], Britain — kicked the bucket February 6, 1804, Northumberland, Pennsylvania, U.S.), English pastor, political scholar, and actual researcher whose work added to progresses in liberal political and strict idea and in exploratory science. He is best associated with his commitment to the science of gases.

Schooling and early vocation

Priestley was naturally introduced to a group of reasonably fruitful fleece material producers in the Calvinist fortress of West Riding, Yorkshire. He entered the Contradicting Foundation at Daventry, Northampton shire, in 1752. Protesters, so named for their reluctance to adjust to the Congregation of Britain, were forestalled by the

Demonstration of Consistency (1662) from entering English colleges. Priestley got brilliant schooling in way of thinking, science, dialects, and writing at Daventry, where he turned into a "irate freethinker" in religion. He revoked the Calvinist tenets of unique sin and reparation, and he embraced a levelheaded Unitarianism that dismissed the Trinity and declared the perfectibility of man.

Somewhere in the range of 1755 and 1761, Priestley served at Needham Market, Suffolk, and at Sandwich, Cheshire. In 1761 he became coach in dialects and writing at the Warrington Foundation, Lancashire. He was appointed a Contradicting clergyman in 1762. That year he wedded Mary Wilkinson, girl of the ironmaster Isaac Wilkinson. They had one little girl and three children.

Work in power

Contraption planned by Joseph Priestley for power age and capacity

Device planned by Joseph Priestley for power age and capacity

Priestley's advantage in science escalated in 1765, when he met the American researcher and legislator Benjamin Franklin, who urged him to distribute The Set of experiences and Current situation with Power, with Unique Trials (1767). In this work, Priestley utilized history to show that logical advancement relied more upon the collection of "new realities" that anybody could find than on the hypothetical bits of knowledge of a couple of men of virtuoso. Priestley's inclination for "realities" over "speculations" in science was reliable with his Contradicting conviction that bias and doctrine of any kind introduced obstructions to individual request and confidential judgment.

This perspective on logical technique molded Priestley's electrical tests, in which he expected the opposite square law of electrical fascination, found that charcoal behaviors power, and noticed the connection among power and compound change. Based on these examinations, in 1766 he was chosen an individual from the Regal Society of London. This line of examination propelled him to create "a bigger field of unique trials" in regions other than power.

The science of gases

Upon his re-visitation of the service at Factory Slope Church, Leeds, in 1767, Priestley started escalated exploratory examinations concerning science. Somewhere in the range of 1772 and 1790, he distributed six volumes of Trials and Perceptions on Various types of Air and in excess of twelve articles in the Regal Society's Philosophical Transactions describing his analyses on gases, or "airs," as they were then called. English pneumatic physicists had recently recognized three sorts of gases: air, carbon dioxide (fixed air), and hydrogen (inflammable air). Priestley integrated a clarification of the science of these gases into the phlogiston hypothesis, as per which flammable substances delivered phlogiston (an irrelevant "standard of inflammability") during consuming.

Priestley found 10 new gases: nitric oxide (nitrous air), nitrogen dioxide (red nitrous fume), nitrous oxide (inflammable nitrous air, later called "snickering gas"), hydrogen chloride (marine corrosive air), smelling salts (basic air), sulfur dioxide (disdainful corrosive air), silicon tetrafluoride (fluor corrosive air), nitrogen (phlogisticated air), oxygen (dephlogisticated air, freely codiscovered via Carl Wilhelm Scheele), and a gas later recognized as carbon monoxide. Priestley's trial achievement came about dominatingly from his capacity to plan shrewd devices and his expertise in their control. He acquired specific eminence for a superior pneumatic box in which, by gathering gases over mercury rather than in water, he had the option to detach and look at gases that were solvent in water. For his work on gases, Priestley was granted the Imperial Society's renowned Copley Award in 1773.

That very year Priestley moved to Cane, Wiltshire, where he filled in as bookkeeper and guide for William Trivial, Lord of Shelburne, and his loved ones. Here he looked for and acquired additional proof supporting his recently found faith in a kind God as opposed to the wrathful Lord of his Calvinist youth. After examining the cycles of vegetation and the "tumult" of oceans and lakes, Priestley imagined the means by which a big-hearted nature reestablished the "normal air" that had been "vitiated and lessened" by such "toxic" processes as ignition and breathe. Aside from fortifying his own otherworldly perspectives, these perceptions informed the photosynthesis tests performed by his counterparts, the Dutch doctor Jan Ingenhousz and the Swiss minister and naturalist Jean Senebier.

Priestley saw his logical interests as reliable with the business and pioneering interests of English Protesters. He embraced the seventeenth century legislator and normal savant Francis Bacon's contention that social advancement required the improvement of a science-based business. This view was supported when he moved to turn into a minister at the New Gathering House in Birmingham in 1780 and turned into an individual from the Lunar Society, a tip top gathering of neighborhood courteous fellows, Dissidents, and industrialists (counting Josiah Wedgwood, Erasmus Darwin, James Watt, and Matthew Boulton), who applied the standards of science and innovation toward the tackling of issues experienced in eighteenth century metropolitan life. At the point when defied by the large number of illnesses that tormented the developing populaces in towns and army bases, Priestley planned a contraption that delivered carbonated water, a blend that he thought would give restorative advantage to victims of scurvy and different fevers. Despite the fact that it eventually demonstrated ineffectual in treating these problems, the "gas gene" that utilized this method later made conceivable the soft drink water industry. Priestley additionally planned the "eudiometer," which was utilized in the overall development for clean change and metropolitan plan to quantify the "virtue" (oxygen content) of air. Contemporary interest in pneumatic medication finished in the brief Pneumatic Foundation, which the doctor and scientist Thomas Beddoes established in Bristol in 1798 to determine the impacts of various "airs" on different normal sicknesses.

The disclosure of oxygen and the synthetic insurgency of Joseph Priestley

Priestley's enduring standing in science is established upon the disclosure he made on August 1, 1774, when he got a dry gas by warming red mercuric oxide. Finding that a candle would consume and that a mouse would flourish in this gas, he referred to it as "dephlogisticated air," in light of the conviction that customary air became immersed with phlogiston once it could never again uphold burning and life. Priestley was not yet certain, nonetheless, that he had found "another types of air." The next October, he went with his supporter, Shelburne, on an excursion through Belgium, Holland, Germany, and France, where in Paris he informed the French scientific expert Antoine Lavoisier how he got the new "air." This gathering between the two researchers was exceptionally huge for the fate of science. Lavoisier promptly rehashed Priestley's analyses and, somewhere in the range of 1775 and 1780, led concentrated examinations from which he determined the rudimentary idea of oxygen, remembered it as the "dynamic" rule in the environment, deciphered its part in burning and breath, and gave it its name. Lavoisier's professions of the movement of oxygen altered science.

All Priestley didn't acknowledge Lavoisier's decisions and proceeded, specifically, to maintain the phlogiston hypothesis. Persuaded that the French physicists were forcing their convictions on mainstream researchers in manners like the Anglican "foundation" of strict and political doctrine, Priestley's Protester leanings reinforced his resistance to Lavoisier's "new arrangement of science." To explain his situation, in 1800 he distributed a thin flyer, Convention of Phlogiston Laid out, and That of the Organization of Water Discredited, which he extended to book length in 1803. The Precept of Phlogiston gave an itemized record of what he imagined to be the exact, hypothetical, and strategic deficiencies of the oxygen hypothesis. Priestley required a patient, modest, exploratory way to deal with God's limitless creation. Science could uphold devotion and freedom provided that it kept away from speculative estimating and energized the perception of God's kindhearted creation. The phlogiston hypothesis was supplanted by Lavoisier's oxidation hypothesis of ignition and breath.

Religious philosophy, educating, and legislative issues

Science was a significant piece of Priestley's "Sane Christianity." In Foundations of Regular and Uncovered Religion (1772-74), he portrayed how he dismissed the "melancholy" Calvinist teachings of the normal debasement of man and the equivocal will of a wrathful God. Priestley utilized clinician and liberal Anglican David Hartley's "precept of relationship of thoughts" to help his view that humankind's perfectibility was the unavoidable outcome of a developing familiarity with man's place in a deterministic arrangement of kindness. In A Set of experiences of the Defilements of Christianity (1782), Priestley guaranteed that the tenets of realism, determinism, and Socinianism (Unitarianism) were reliable with an objective perusing of the Book of scriptures. He demanded that Jesus Christ was a simple man who taught the revival of the body instead of the everlasting status of a nonexistent soul.

In 1765 he was granted a LL.D. from the College of Edinburgh for his instructive and scholarly achievements at Warrington. These remembered his works for Hypothesis of Language and Widespread Punctuation (1762), An Exposition on a Course of Liberal Training for Common and Dynamic Life (1765), and Talks on History and General Strategy (ready at Warrington however not distributed until 1788). Priestley utilized "the convention of relationship of thoughts" to help his perspectives on language, history, and schooling also. Specifically, he based what he considered to be the right utilization of language on the standard relationship of thoughts. He likewise utilized instructing procedures that depended on the encounters of his understudies and were intended to set them up for a down to earth life.

Priestley joined hypothesis and practice in his work in legislative issues. In 1767 he became associated with the Protester's public battle against the Test and Enterprise Act (1661) that limited their common and political freedoms. In

An Article on the Main Standards of Government (1768), he contended that logical advancement and human perfectibility required the right to speak freely of discourse, love, and training. As a defender of free enterprise financial matters, created by the Scottish thinker Adam Smith, Priestley looked to restrict the job of government and to assess its viability exclusively with regards to the government assistance of the person. The English financial specialist and pioneer behind utilitarianism Jeremy Bentham recognized that Priestley's powerful book enlivened the expression used to portray his own development, "the best bliss of the best number."

Strife and exile

The English press and government declared that Priestley's help, along with that of his companion, the ethical savant Richard Cost, of the American and French Unrests was "subversive." On July 14, 1791, the "Congregation and-Lord crowd" annihilated Priestley's home and research center. Priestley and his family withdrew to the security of Value's assemblage at Hackney, close to London. Priestley later started educating at New School, Oxford, and shielded his enemy of English government sees in Letters to One side Decent Edmund Burke (1791).

Priestley's guard failed to receive any notice as the moderate response to the French Upset escalated in Britain. In 1794 he escaped to the US, where he found a type of government that was "generally passable." His most popular writing in the US, Letters to the Occupants of Northumberland (1799), turned out to be essential for the conservative reaction to the Federalists. Priestley passed on at Northumberland, Pennsylvania, grieved and respected by Thomas Jefferson, the third leader of the US.

Nitrous oxide has been utilized restoratively as a sedative and a pain relieving for over 100 years. The sedative impact is believed to be intervened fundamentally by the reversible restraint of the N-methyl-d-aspartate sort of glutamate receptors bringing about hindrance of excitatory glutamatergic neurotransmission. Nitrous oxide applies it pain relieving impacts by means of enactment of opioidergic neurons. Most critical human openness to nitrous oxide happens in clinical settings either by restorative organization or as accidental openness. Word related openness limits are suggested where nitrous oxide is controlled regularly to patients. Nitrous oxide has been utilized as a sporting medication, and ongoing maltreatment makes caused unsafe neurologic impacts and demise. Naturally, nitrous oxide is an intense ozone harming substance delivered principally from rural exercises.

Nitrous oxide is the new and most significant guilty party harming the ozone layer (Fig. 18.5). It is the biggest reason for ozone layer consumption. This is on the grounds that CFCs and numerous different gases that harm the ozone layer were restricted by the Montreal Convention (MP), and at present their environmental fixations have decreased considerably. Nitrous oxide isn't limited by the MP, so while the degree of other ozone layer exhausting substances (ODS) are declining, nitrous oxide levels are expanding. These effects are supposed to turn out to be more serious, except if purposeful endeavors are made to diminish emanations.

Nitrous oxide and nitric oxide spending plans

Adjusting nitrous oxide sources and sinks to foster a worldwide nitrous oxide spending plan (Table 20.2) has been difficult for specialists. Soils from regular and farming biological systems represent the greater part of worldwide nitrous oxide discharges. The excess nitrous oxide is generally delivered in the seas, by petroleum derivative ignition and modern cycles, and from biomass consuming (e.g., backwoods fires). Nitrous oxide is eliminated from the air for the most part by photochemical responses in stratosphere, which is a sluggish cycle: the typical home season of a N2O particle is over 100 years. Soil microorganisms can eliminate limited quantities of environmental nitrous oxide under certain conditions, however this is typically offset a lot more prominent paces of nitrous oxide creation.

A moderately predictable yearly expansion in environmental N2O gathering (~4 TG year-1 of N2O-N) has happened throughout recent many years. This noticed increment concurs with the contrast between our worldwide appraisals of sources (~17 Tg N year-1) and sinks of nitrous oxide (13 TG N year-1; Table 20.2). Consequently, at the worldwide scale, our "base up" appraisals of nitrous oxide discharges from numerous sources and evacuation pathways roughly match "top down" perceptions of air nitrous oxide. In any case, at more limited sizes these evaluations can differ significantly. One generally involved approach for assessing base up outflows includes emanations factors, for which a given part of nitrogen inputs (e.g., 1% of manufactured manure) or environment nitrogen pools (e.g., 1% harvest deposits) is anticipated to be let out of soil as nitrous oxide. The US Corn Belt is a district of escalated horticulture that gets enormous contributions of responsive nitrogen from manure and natural nitrogen obsession. Hierarchical estimations in this area show a lot more noteworthy barometrical nitrous oxide fixations than can be represented by soil nitrous oxide emanations assessed from discharges factors. Little streams that channel from farming watersheds can create exceptionally high nitrous oxide emanations from DE nitrification and could consequently represent part of this missing source (Griffins et al., 2017). Nonetheless, long haul estimations have additionally shown that high nitrous oxide discharges from agrarian soils likewise add to territorial misjudges naturally outflows factors (Gillette et al., 2018). Working on our ability to gauge nitrous oxide outflows at the site and provincial scales stays a functioning area of exploration that is basic to illuminate strategy and the executives for diminishing the emanations of this strong ozone harming substance.

As opposed to nitrous oxide, nitric oxide is an exceptionally fleeting compound in the environment (hours-weeks), and its financial plan is considerably more earnestly to gauge than for nitrous oxide. In light of extrapolation from field estimations of soil nitric oxide discharges, worldwide nitric oxide emanations from soil normal 21 Tg NO-N year-1 except for with enormous vulnerability spreading over 4–10 Tg NO-N year-1 (Davidson and Kimberlee, 1997).

Nitrous Oxide Creation

Nitrous oxide (N2O) is a powerful ozone depleting substance that has likewise been ensnared in stratospheric ozone exhaustion (Capone, 1991). The environmental stock of N2O is by and by expanding, so there is a recharged interest in the marine biological system as an expected wellspring of N2O. Nitrous oxide is a follow gas in seawater with regular focuses going from 5 to 50 nmol L–1. Groupings of N2O in maritime surface waters are for the most part in slight overabundance of air immersion, suggesting both a nearby source and a supported sea to-environment transition. Normally there is a mid-water (500-1000 m) top in N2O focus that harmonizes with the broke down oxygen least. At these middle of the road water profundities, N2O can surpass 300% immersion comparative with barometrical balance. The two most plausible wellsprings of N2O in the sea are nitrification and DE nitrification, despite the fact that to date measuring the overall commitment of every pathway for most habitats has been troublesome. Isotopic estimations of nitrogen and oxygen could demonstrate priceless in such manner. Since the different nitrogen cycle responses are interconnected, changes in the pace of any one interaction will probably affect the others. For instance, determination for N2-fixing organic entities as a result of residue statement or conscious iron preparation would expand the neighborhood NH4+ stock and lead to speed up paces of nitrification and, subsequently, could prompt improved N2O creation in the surface sea and transition to the environment.

Nitrous Oxide

Nitrous oxide (N2O) makes up roughly 5% of U.S. GWP-weighted ozone depleting substance outflows. Discharges gauges for N2O are more dubious than those for either carbon dioxide or methane. Assessed nitrous oxide emanations have been generally steady during the 1990s, without an undeniable pattern. The reexamined appraisals of nitrous oxide emanations incorporate one huge class of sources and two little classes (see Figure 9.5). Agribusiness is the chief source, overwhelmed by discharges from nitrogen treatment of farming soils. Auxiliary N2O outflows from nitrogen in farming spillover into streams and waterways have been consolidated. Engine vehicles outfitted with exhaust systems likewise emanate huge measures of N2O.9 Synthetic cycles, fuel burning, and wastewater treatment plants are similarly little producers of N2O.

Nitrous oxide (N2O), generally known as snickering gas, is the most elevated nitrogen-containing compound in the lower environment. Its true capacity for warming per unit atom is multiple times that of carbon dioxide. It is likewise one of the ozone depleting substances restricted by the Kyoto Convention. The normal wellspring of nitrous oxide is fundamentally the arrival of marine and tropical woods. Anthropogenic sources are principally agrarian creation processes, modern creation, and animal's outflows, representing multiple/3 of the all-out emanations. Nitrous oxide must be disposed of by sluggish photolysis in the stratosphere, and subsequently has a long lifetime of around long term in the air. The grouping of nitrous oxide has been kept up with at around 270 pub for over 1000 years before the modern transformation yet expanded at a pace of 0.2%-0.3% each year after that. By 2008, the worldwide normal centralization of nitrous oxide has reached 321.8 ppbv.

Nitrous Oxide (N2O)

Nitrous oxide is another significant ozone depleting substance that is available in raised focuses in estuarine conditions. As of now, N2O is liable for around 5-6% of the anthropogenic nursery impact and is expanding in the environment at a pace of around 0.25% each year. Notwithstanding, the job of estuaries in the worldwide financial plan of the gas has just been tended to as of late.

Nitrous oxide is created fundamentally as a transitional during both nitrification (the oxidation of ammonium to nitrate) and DE nitrification (the decrease of nitrate, through nitrite and N2O, to nitrogen gas), in spite of the fact that creation by dissimulator nitrate decrease to ammonium is additionally conceivable. In estuaries, nitrification and DE nitrification are both remembered to be significant sources. Factors, for example, the oxygen level in the estuary and the nitrate and ammonium convergences of the water can impact which pathway is prevailing, with DE nitrification ruling at extremely low, however non-zero, oxygen fixations. Nitrous oxide fixations are regularly most noteworthy in the segments of the estuary nearest to the waterways, and lessening with distance downstream. Various specialists have announced nitrous oxide maxima in estuarine waters at low salinities (<5-10 on the PSU scale), yet this isn't generally the situation. The turbidity greatest has been accounted for to be the site of most extreme nitrification (probably in light of expanded home time for microbes joined to suspended particulate matter, joined with raised substrate (oxygen and ammonium)).

Table 2 presents an outline of the information distributed for level of immersion and air-estuary transition of nitrous oxide from different estuaries, which are all situated in

Europe and North America. Fixations are generally over that anticipated from air-ocean harmony, and assessments of transitions range from 0.01 μmol m−2 h−1 to 5 μmol m−2 h−1. Vivacity isn't significant for nitrous oxide since it is substantially more solvent than methane. Analysts have assessed the size of the worldwide estuarine hotspot for N2O in light of transitions from individual estuaries duplicated by the worldwide region involved by estuaries to go from 0.22 Tg N2O y−1 to 5.7 Tg y−1 relying upon the attributes of the waterways contemplated. Free gauges in light of financial plans of nitrogen contribution to waterways, suspicions about the small amount of inorganic nitrogen species eliminated by nitrification or DE nitrification, and the fragmentary 'yield' of nitrous oxide creation during these cycles demonstrate that nitrous oxide transitions to the air from estuaries is around.

The sporting utilization of nitrous oxide (N2O; snickering gas) has to a great extent extended as of late. Albeit coincidental utilization of nitrous oxide barely goals any wellbeing harm, tricky or weighty utilization of nitrous oxide can prompt serious unfriendly impacts. Amsterdam care focuses saw that Moroccan-Dutch youthful grown-ups revealed neurological side effects, including extreme loss of motion, because of risky nitrous oxide use. In this subjective exploratory review, thirteen youthful grown-up Moroccan-Dutch unreasonable nitrous oxide clients were evaluated. The determinants of hazardous nitrous oxide use in this ethnic gathering are talked about, including their low therapy interest as for nitrous oxide misuse related clinical mental issues. Intentions in utilizing nitrous oxide are to alleviate weariness, to search out unwinding with companions and to smother psychosocial stress and negative contemplations. Different thought processes are discouragement, segregation and struggle with companions or guardians. The no culture encompassing substance use — question, disgrace and macho culture — disappoints opportune clinical/mental treatment of Moroccan-Dutch tricky nitrous oxide clients. It is prescribed to involve powerhouses in media crusades with the expect to diminish the dangers of weighty nitrous oxide use and further develop treatment access. Outreach youth laborers can likewise assume a significant part in persuading socially disengaged clients to look for clinical or potentially mental assistance.

Pervasiveness of Nitrous Oxide Use

Sporting nitrous oxide use is characterized as less than ten nitrous oxide inflatables per occasion or each month [2]. As per the Worldwide Medication Study [4,5], nitrous oxide has turned into the seventh most involved sporting medication in the UK with a last year use commonness of 21% in 2013 (normal age: 24.3 years). The 2016/17 Wrongdoing Overview for Britain and Ribs announced that among the 16-24 year old subjects, the last year commonness of nitrous oxide use was 9.3% (guys, 11.1%; females, 7.4%) [6]. The Worldwide Medication Overview 2016 detailed that last year use in the Netherlands was 33% versus 38% and 23.7% in the Unified Realm [4]. To be sure, in the Netherlands, nitrous oxide is acquiring prevalence in both optional school understudies [7] and everybody [8], particularly among youthful grown-ups and the people who are exceptionally taught [9]. In excess of a fourth of the understudies (30%) of post-optional professional schooling detailed that they had involved nitrous oxide in 2019 with 8% in the previous month.

Students with a non-Western transient foundation have more involvement in the utilization of nitrous oxide than understudies without a traveler foundation [9]. A new study among Dutch youths (14-18 years of age) verifies these outcomes as nitrous oxide use was related with a non-Dutch ethnic foundation (OR = 2.10), lower schooling levels (OR = 1.88) and hard-core boozing (OR = 2.49) [11]. Last year and last month utilization of nitrous oxide among Dutch individuals with a non-Western transient foundation (3.6% and 1.2%, separately) is higher than among those with a Dutch foundation (2.5% and 0.8%, separately).

The greater part (77%) of nitrous oxide clients knew nothing about the medication's hurtful impacts [5] and accepted that the medication was protected on account of its lawful status [2]. Nonetheless, the legitimate status for generally youthful grown-up "party clients" is unessential in their choice to utilize nitrous oxide [2]. Because of the rising sporting utilization of nitrous oxide throughout recent years, including overall [12], a lawful restriction is being considered to counter this. Until further notice, nitrous oxide has been dependent upon the Products Act in the Netherlands (since July 2016). In France, a few towns have proactively prohibited the offer of the gas to under 18-year-olds, and drives are in progress to boycott the deal to minors cross country.

Unfriendly Impacts of Nitrous Oxide Use

The recurrence of nitrous oxide use fluctuates with the biggest gathering involving nitrous oxide on more than one occasion in the previous year (45%), while 16% did so in excess of multiple times [16]. Coincidental utilization of nitrous oxide is scarcely, or not by any stretch of the imagination, related with significant harm to wellbeing. Every now and again revealed incidental effects are cerebral pain, unsteadiness, swooning, unintentional falls and shivering of hands and feet. Nitrous oxide instigated diligent deadness/tinging (fringe neuropathy; paresthesia) in hands or feet is a portion subordinate neurological impact with relentless deadness in 4.3% of last year clients.

Notwithstanding, the wellbeing harm of nitrous oxide, including its reliance risk, increments quickly with day to day use in higher everyday portions; once in a while many cartridges were breathed in each day [18]. Particularly after the development of bigger nitrous oxide tanks (2-Kg tanks) in 2017-2018, the quantity of serious neurological objections expanded [19]. Following escalated use (10-20 inflatables or all the more everyday), serious neurological confusions, for example, myelopathy and summed up demyelinating polyneuropathy can happen because of nitrous oxide instigated lack of vitamin B12. These difficulties are typically reversible and can commonly be settled through vitamin B12 supplementation (infusions), however the neurological recuperation might be hindered of even inadequate on the off chance that patients keep on utilizing nitrous oxide [26].

The Medication Occurrences Screen enlisted a restricted however expanding number of episodes including nitrous oxide (in 2018: 51 reports; 0.8% of all medication episodes) [9]. In 2019, the Dutch Toxic substance Community (NVIC) got 128 reports of wellbeing grumblings in individuals matured 13 and over after sporting utilization of nitrous oxide. Neurological protests were accounted for in about 33% of the reports, which demonstrated (ongoing) maltreatment of enormous amounts. In 42 out of 78 emergency clinics reached by the Dutch Nervous system specialists' Affiliation, 64 youthful grown-ups (mean age: 22 years) with a halfway spinal line injury following nitrous oxide use had been treated in the beyond two years (2018-2019) [27], yet the genuine number of casualties is accepted to be more noteworthy. The new expansion in nitrous oxide related traffic episodes is one more place of concern [9].

Moroccan-Dutch Youthful Grown-ups

Throughout the course of recent years, the quantity of nitrous oxide-related patients at the Reade restoration focus, the crisis division (OLVG emergency clinic, Amsterdam, The Netherlands) and habit care (Jellied) has consistently expanded. Albeit this has not yet been investigated and careful figures are not accessible, it includes a few dozen youthful grown-up clients every year (for the most part in their twenties), most of whom have a Moroccan transient foundation. For that reason this explorative review zeroed in explicitly on Moroccan-Dutch youth. In the following segment, a short outline is given of the conviction, substance use, wellbeing and youth culture in this gathering, in light of the fact that these gave off an impression of being determinant of nitrous oxide misuse.

A huge part (94%) of Moroccan-Dutch, including those having a place with the second era [28], see themselves as strict yet non-rehearsing Muslims [29], while the strict view of their folks is more grounded than that of the youthful grown-ups. Especially among youthful grown-up Muslims, Islamic convictions frequently have areas of strength for an impact by the way they see shared connections and (on the web) interpersonal organizations [33]. Contrasted with the Dutch, Moroccan-Dutch by and large have more nearby and family ties, more homogeneous organizations and their standards and values more moderate. For the Moroccan-Dutch, religion assumes a larger part throughout everyday life, resistance toward "present day" conduct is more restricted and they are likewise less happy with their lives than the Dutch [34].

Drug Use in an Untouchable Culture

Ethnic minorities, similar to the Moroccan-Dutch people group, live somewhat more frequently in socially denied regions and are all the more frequently less taught and jobless; factors related with hazardous liquor and medication use [35]. Maybe significantly more pertinent as for liquor and substance addiction by Muslims is that it is important for Muslim no culture: the utilization of substances is "haram" (evil). Thusly, youthful grown-up Muslims might find it challenging to direct their drinking conduct, which can prompt extreme liquor utilization, particularly in tricky home circumstances (especially in private youth care) [36]. Contrasted with Turkish-Dutch, Moroccan-Dutch beverage 1.7 times more liquor and multiple times more inordinate liquor (15.4% and 5.3%, separately). Moroccan-Dutch in Amsterdam have an expanded gamble of liquor misuse (OR = 2.25; 95% CI: 1.44-3.53) and normal consumers of Moroccan plunge have an essentially higher gamble of creating "gorge" drinking and liquor reliance than standard consumers in other ethnic minority bunches [39]. As for pot, dangerous use is more normal among clients with a non-Western transient foundation than their Dutch friends (33% and 17%, separately) [9].

Hazardous utilization of medications may likewise emerge from different individual, sociocultural elements (unfortunate social help from family or companions) and additionally mental variables (low confidence, minimization, segregation, derision, forlornness, weariness) [40]. The low confidence may likewise come about because of assimilating issues connected with poor parental help, parent-kid struggle, school/peer (being exhausted) and the young adult's apparent separation, as seen among foreigner youths in the Netherlands [41]. Youthful Moroccan grown-ups in the Netherlands frequently feel victimized predominantly based on their religion and Muslim personality [42] and don't consider completely fledged [43], and feel trashed, separated and prohibited [42]. A new precise survey showed that segregation was related with weighty and perilous drinking, especially inside pressure and adapting structures [44]. Moreover, slander of medication reliance can thwart individuals' quest for treatment. Abstaining from looking for help or potentially denying a (serious) close to home issue can likewise heighten issues. That reality that mental diseases are many times no inside Moroccan families is one more mark of concern [47]. For sure, youthful grown-ups with a Moroccan and Turkish foundation are underrepresented in normal youth psychological well-being care: about portion of what can be generally anticipated demographically.

In this subjective exploratory review, we had the one of a kind chance to meet with youthful Moroccan-Dutch weighty clients of nitrous oxide determined to recognize determinants of hazardous nitrous oxide use. This is one of a kind since this gathering is hesitant to share their contemplations about substance use, which for them is interwoven with disgrace.

Techniques

Acquiring admittance to dangerous nitrous oxide clients beyond institutional settings is troublesome. This issue is especially intense for nitrous oxide as these clients seldom come into contact with therapy administrations and those that do are probably not going to be illustrative of the bigger populace of clients. The enlistment system didn't create a genuinely irregular example, essentially because of weighty obstruction by sensations of disgrace among this gathering of hazardous nitrous oxide clients. In view of prior signals in the examination field, we picked to carry out our groundwork inside the New-West locale of Amsterdam, where generally numerous Moroccan-Dutch individuals reside. In this area mostly Moroccan-Dutch youthful grown-ups show tricky nitrous oxide use, which was our essential consideration measure.

The gathering of risky nitrous oxide clients comprised of two gatherings: seven youthful grown-ups (5 men, 2 ladies; 19-28 years) who were in clinical or short term treatment (Reade and Jellied) for their dangerous utilization of nitrous oxide and six youthful grown-ups (5 men, 1 lady; 19-22 years) who vigorously utilize nitrous oxide, however who are not in treatment. The clients who were not in treatment (N = 6) were selected by youth laborers in the New-West area who applied the compounding procedure. The other gathering (N = 7) were enlisted by patients' professional during the admission in the clinical and short term treatment communities. All interviewees had a Moroccan transient foundation (matured 18-29 years) and lived with their folks/sister.

A rundown of points were drawn up, covering inquiries concerning their utilization profile (recurrence, portion), thought processes of purpose, mindfulness about wellbeing chances, impacts experienced and their reaction to them and determinants of looking for help or not. This rundown (cf. Table 1) filled in as a rule for the (top to bottom) interview. Before the top to bottom meeting, the seven members who were in treatment were evaluated for one hour about issues, like childhood, confidence, family, companions, training, work, going out and their assumptions for what's in store. The inside and out interview of roughly 2.5 h was principally centered around their concerns with nitrous oxide and extra inquiries were posed to about thought processes in use, recurrence and measurements, wellbeing grievances and utilization of online entertainment. Besides, data was gathered about the (no) culture around liquor and medication use, their impression of wellbeing dangers and care arrangement and why they entered medical care at such a late stage. The six youngsters who didn't get treatment were evaluated for roughly 1.5 h with questions that depended on a more limited rundown of points. All respondents demanded that the meetings not be recorded. The members got a EUR 50 voucher as pay for the meeting. The experts were consulted for around 1.5 h about the living climate, the social space of neighborhood youth from various ethnic foundations and the gamble variables to which they are uncovered.

The hazardous utilization of nitrous oxide was a delicate subject for every single youthful grown-up; they were not anxious to talk about it and some were dubious or embarrassed to examine their traditions. They expressed that through their accounts they would have liked to make youthful grown-ups more mindful of the wellbeing takes a chance with that nitrous oxide can cause. The youthful grown-ups talked with are social Muslims, where confidence is significant, however they don't rehearse their confidence (no imploring or visiting the mosque). Some are particular Muslims who consistently take part in the social and ceremonial practices, however not often. A few respondents featured the twofold norm in disposition toward drug use; that it is all the more not entirely obvious and more acknowledged for men to utilize drugs than ladies.

Beginning with Nitrous Oxide Use

In their extra time, the youthful grown-ups are in many cases somewhere else other than at home as the normally little houses in which they live bear the cost of little security. There is somewhat little family pay as the dads frequently have low-talented work, while the moms primarily do the housework. The youthful grown-ups themselves follow or followed professional preparation and began working in the wake of having gotten their expert confirmation. A couple have exited partially through and are jobless. A few said they have a liberal pay for their age; a few youngsters were unclear about how they brought in cash yet implied that they are engaged with unlawful deals (nitrous oxide and cocaine) and benefit well from it. One respondent (male, 22 years of age), who is likewise selling nitrous oxide, has youngsters from the local who convey nitrous oxide tanks to clients for him. This image is reliable with the tales of respondents, of whom half report they have collected obligation (counting medical coverage, understudy obligation or obligations to relatives) because of inordinate nitrous oxide use. At last, subsequent to having spoken with youth and social laborers in the field, it would be not difficult to get the feeling that nitrous oxide is famous just with minimized youth in road societies. Be that as it may, other youthful grown-ups who additionally dwell in these areas never had contact with youth work or the police, have finished a training and looked for a decent job. The discussions show that they experienced nitrous oxide by means of different courses (companions, associates at work or in the nightlife circuit).

The respondents' interest was frequently set off by the "publicity" around nitrous oxide. Cool craftsmen began singing decidedly about inflatables in cuts, a few companions had nitrous oxide whippets (little steel cartridges of 10 cc), and young ladies possibly needed to come to your party when there was nitrous oxide, neighborhood shops began to publicize and companions began exchanging with nitrous oxide through virtual entertainment. Most youngsters began utilizing nitrous oxide when they were underage (15-17 years of age). In all cases, this was finished in gatherings: during a school trip, after school at somebody's home, along with young ladies and different companions in a lodging, a shisha relax, carport, park, an ocean side tent or holiday in Morocco, as a respondent actually recalled well. "My most memorable time was in an underground bar in Tangier where we utilized expands along for certain companions. Nitrous oxide isn't permitted in Morocco, yet somebody from the Netherlands had snuck in a freight load and ensured that traditions would deliberately ignore. There was limitless nitrous oxide at that party, and I involved a great deal of inflatables interestingly. The servers were constantly filling inflatables through a whipped cream needle. I didn't need to pay anything since us young ladies never need to pay for their beverages and inflatables. We feel that is ordinary. That is the manner in which it goes" (Lady, 27 years of age).

One male respondent (19 years of age) said that the utilization of nitrous oxide inflatables began when he was exhausted with companions. The environment is promptly more tomfoolery and there are a considerable amount of folks in the space who make it happen. In this way, it isn't so exceptional. Despite the fact that he saw individuals freaking out. Youngsters who don't have anything to do with it leave naturally when it is swell time. One respondent recalls when he was in a recreation area with a gathering. One companion out of nowhere appeared with a case of nitrous oxide cartridges. He was a beginner and had never plastered, smoked or drank liquor previously. "I would have rather not from the beginning, however when I saw that it fulfilled them, I likewise needed to attempt an inflatable. I felt shivering in my mind. It was a magnificent inclination" (Man, 19 years of age). A 17-year-elderly person accepted her most memorable nitrous oxide swell from a fuel tank. During that period, she invested a ton of energy with a companion whose guardians were much of the time away in Dubai. "There was normally nitrous oxide, a 2-Kg tank you know. We were four young ladies. They previously had insight with inflatables. Whenever I first just did four. It was a great, drifting inclination" (Lady, 19 years of age). At the point when school shut (because of

Coronavirus) she began utilizing pretty much consistently with a sweetheart where young men generally accompanied new tanks. "I never needed to pay for it. It was consistently there."

Drug Consumptions

The possibility that nitrous oxide is modest may apply to sporting clients who sometimes use inflatables, however not too risky clients who think as far as 2-Kg tanks costing EUR 40-50 (for around 125-150 inflatables) and in the interim have utilized many such tanks or spent EUR 30,000-50,000. One respondent actually has an obligation of EUR 11,000 to his sister, while one more said: " I breathed in nitrous oxide worth 30,000 euros, bringing about a spinal rope injury." Conversely, the ladies talked with said when they are going out, they seldom need to pay for their entry, liquor or nitrous oxide inflatables, which thus now and again prompts mental tension for some of them when the "liberal" provider begins making references about receiving something consequently. Discussions with ladies, stories course, affirm past discoveries in Amsterdam, about purported "swell prostitutes" who engage in sexual relations with young fellows in return free of charge nitrous oxide; these young men are alluded to buy them as "Jacks". A few ladies scrutinize young men's twofold norms. They grumble that young ladies anticipate that they should need to "orchestrate" the nitrous oxide, and yet, celebrating without young ladies is less tomfoolery. "Thus, if you need to dial back the utilization of nitrous oxide in young men, you need to persuade the young ladies not to hit up those nitrous oxide parties", said a lady (18 years of age).

Insight and Involvement in Liquor and Medications

All members revealed that according to a strict perspective, liquor and medication use is marked extremely negative (haram) in their family, and that this no subject is scarcely at any point examined at home. Except for one respondent (Lady, 19 years of age) whose father is as of now not a Muslim (mother is). "The mosque cautions about the mistakes of psyche brought about by drug use. It takes you from following the way. You get mentally trapped and it creates turmoil" (Man, 29 years of age). As indicated by one respondent, drug use isn't really deterred for wellbeing reasons, but since the Heavenly Quran basically dismisses the utilization of intoxicants. "I've forever been informed it's illegal in my religion, generally my folks could utilize it as well" (Man, 22 years of age). Another man said that his mom once made a correlation with stick sniffers in Morocco and that youngsters in the Netherlands would face a similar outcome as the unfortunate road kids in Morocco. One respondent (Man, 19 years of age) said that he was cautioned about drugs since the beginning: "You shouldn't do whatever annihilates your body". At the point when he was 13 years of age, his more seasoned sibling intrigued on him that he ought to never acknowledge a joint from another person, since then he would as of now not be lucid while supplicating. It is additionally striking that most youths in auxiliary school (counting optional professional training) said that they had never been shown about liquor and medications. It might try and happen that the dad utilizes pot, yet prohibits his kids to utilize it, as two ladies have encountered. "Drugs are an off limits with us devotees since they obliterate your body. However, clearly this standard doesn't have any significant bearing to men. My dad smokes hash consistently. That is a twofold norm" (Lady, 27 years of age).

The respondents frequently detailed that they don't smoke at home or drink liquor keeping in mind their folks. However, numerous respondents have utilized liquor and marijuana. A minority experienced MDMA or cocaine eventually yet really like to maintain it mystery to stay away from clashes at home, and devise reasons and methodologies to stay out of contentions. As youngsters progress in years, they find the nightlife where individuals drink and use drugs, so the probability of struggles increments. In the phase of immaturity, they begin to make their own arrangements, regardless of whether medications are disallowed. Whoever gets back home with a tobacco or liquor smell can anticipate the rage of the dad of the house. "Nitrous oxide is legitimate, and your folks don't know since it is scentless, and the impacts are not apparent. Perhaps it will decrease the aggravation of your lie to your folks a piece" (Man, 26 years of age).

Some say they don't keep the guidelines and decide on a showdown and get back inebriated or stoned. "My folks' lessons might have helped initially, yet as you age, it makes you poo" (Man, 19 years of age). A lady (18 years of age) no longer needs to act fraudulently and has let her folks know that she smokes, in some cases beverages and utilizations nitrous oxide. Regarding their folks' limitations, some show up at home after the guardians are snoozing or choose to rest somewhere else. A respondent who began to find the nightlife remained over with her Dutch sweetheart all together not to humiliate her folks and to keep up with her own power. One more respondent liked to go through the night with a "neighborhood addict" or in his own vehicle in an unwanted parking spot. He educated us that it's an exercise in futility to talk since it is haram and essentially not permitted. They realize that he once in a while drinks liquor. "When I got back home alcoholic at 5.30 toward the beginning of the day. I was late and I had plastered a ton and got into a gigantic debate with my dad. As discipline, I needed to remain inside for a couple of days. So keeping in mind my folks, I like to remain away when I've been drinking" (Man, 21 years of age).

While their folks are frequently emphatically against drugs, the respondents' companions are more open minded. One respondent (Lady, 19 years of age) told how she began trying different things with marijuana inside a gathering of companions among breaks and after school. Youngsters additionally discuss parties in shisha lounges, lodgings, clubs and confidential homes organized via landowners with associations with nitrous oxide merchants. Communicating with companions of various identities in your extra time can work with assimilation, so these youngsters become more lenient toward drugs. On respondent (Man 22, years of age) says that he didn't drink a lot of liquor. His last time was a half year prior on New Year's Eve. In any case, he additionally understood that "the tissue is frail" when he begins drinking. "We then request huge jugs of vodka that we will wave around (snickers). By purchasing a container you show that you hit the nail on the head. Regardless of whether you just have 50 euros, you actually purchase that jug. You get it?" He finds it troublesome not to drink since he resides in the Netherlands where liquor is so natural to get. On the off chance that the principles at home are so severe, he's considerably more headed to rebel. The Dutch are open minded and more tolerating of liquor use. Moroccans, be that as it may, don't figure out how to drink from companions or relatives thus once they begin drinking can't restrict their liquor consumption he says. "At the point when we drink and do inflatables, it is much of the time out of an issue and not really for no particular reason" (Man, 21 years of age).

Enjoying something, yet in addition feeling remorseful and awful simultaneously prompts disarray, strain and uncertainty about what your identity is and who you need to be. The members revealed that they should continuously "switch" from parent culture to school and road culture, as well as the other way around, and each time assume an alternate part. "It takes a great deal of energy assuming you need to turn that button on and off constantly" said one respondent. (Female, 27 years of age). Another lady (19 years of age) has been informed a few times by her dad that she is a prostitute in the event that she doesn't get back home on time. Pressures some of the time run so intense that she yearns for a spot somewhere else. Youngsters frequently feel misjudged by their folks and can't act naturally in the distressing, manly road culture. In road culture, young men impact again with "ladylike" school culture which animates self-articulation and self-advancement. A "bungle" among instructors and understudies can be unfortunate for school execution and consequently propagate a negative mental self-portrait. As per a few youngsters, this to a great extent affects the manner in which they carry on with their life. Because of strict (Moroccan) childhood, which deters substance use, Moroccan-Dutch youthful grown-ups use liquor and medications less frequently than their local Dutch companions. In like manner, the youthful grown-ups talked with additionally rarely drink liquor, with a periodic exception for some. Pot is all the more generally utilized, particularly in road societies, while cocaine and rapture are seldom utilized, with a couple of exemptions. Notwithstanding, nitrous oxide is an exemption that obviously affirms the standard.

Thought processes in Nitrous Oxide Use

The sporting utilization of nitrous oxide (for instance occasion, birthday, nightlife), ended up being more tricky among the respondents who battle most with their Moroccan culture in Dutch society and experience the ill effects of a character emergency. Detailed intentions (set factors as per the Zinberg model; cf. Conversation) to utilize nitrous oxide incorporate to keep away from weariness, look for unwinding, and decrease pressure and to stop enthusiastic negative contemplations. The tension of working, considering, keeping up with kinships and misleading your folks is distressing. Nitrous oxide can give solace through impermanent unwinding and help and appears to offer the main relief. One respondent (Man, 19 years of age) said: "I was so bustling in my mind that I could unwind with inflatables during the end of the week." Others notice vacancy, forlornness, gloom, segregation, clashes with companions or guardians, a deficiency of acknowledgment and appreciation, a powerlessness to communicate sentiments and feeling of dread toward disappointment. "You generally get the inclination that you are a peasant," a respondent (Man, 26 years of age) told us. He said that even his Dutch mother by marriage has little to no faith in him since he is a Muslim. A 19-year-elderly person lets us know that inflatables gave her a cheerful inclination first and foremost, however she gradually understood that it was likewise a departure from issues. The more she began utilizing the more she experienced amnesia and focus issues. "I hushed up about saying: this is my last inflatable, this is the last inflatable, this is…. Nitrous oxide makes everything poop. It makes you foolish. Yet, what did I need to lose?" A few respondents even saw different clients outperforming their own utilization during occasion periods and the Coronavirus emergency. It is a risky time, they said, on the grounds that youngsters don't have the foggiest idea where they stand and how lengthy it will take before they can return to school, play sports and go on siestas. Weariness set in. "Crown aggravated the issue. I got into an emergency about what my identity was. I'm Moroccan indeed, however I in all actuality do feel stuck between two universes. You don't actually well with anybody. That is the reason I needed to get out of the real world" (Lady, 19 years of age). Another lady (27 years of age) says that she can remain in charge with inflatables. One benefit is that guardians don't take note. "They don't see it in you, it doesn't possess an aroma like liquor or tobacco. You can simply continue to talk. They don't see your students. No one takes note. Furthermore, that is the reason it's so hazardous, on the grounds that it's alluring. And yet, you feel remorseful."

The Development of Hazardous Use

With the appearance of the enormous 2-Kg nitrous oxide tanks on the medication market (just EUR 40) around 2017-2018, the utilization of nitrous oxide expanded quickly. Youthful business visionaries — they were likewise impressive clients themselves — began a rewarding business zeroed in on the rising interest from their own areas. Conveyance administrations worked every minute of every day so that orders could likewise be filled around evening time. Nitrous oxide is most likely the principal drug (with the exception of pot) that Moroccan-Dutch individuals offer to one another, which might make sense of the quick spread in the local locations of New-West. A few youths began to find the ordinary nightlife of clubs, shisha lounges and late get-togethers and in equal, inn parties where companions could assemble utilizing nitrous oxide consistently. "Everything was guiltless up to the place of those large tanks," one respondent (29 years of age) told us. He could now siphon huge inflatables consistently and felt as was he "caught in a pattern of purpose without interference and high constantly."

Two ladies revealed that they consistently wound up in confidential houses (10-15 individuals) where 10-Kg tanks were conveyed relentless throughout the end of the week. All respondents began utilizing more when they changed to the bigger tanks, which were simpler to work and, from certain perspectives, were additionally more secure to utilize. "In the event that you can get it that simple, it can't be unsafe, can it? Definitely the public authority could have acted quite a while in the past and restricted the medication?" one respondent pronounced (Man 26 years of age). The utilization of Nitrous accelerated enormously with the appearance of 2-Kg tanks available. Not least due to usability. "You open that tap and you can explode however many inflatables as you need", one client (Man, 22 years of age) says. He giggles about the quarrel he had before with those dated whippets. "Each time placing a whippet in the holder, turning it on, fitting gas into the needle, expand over the valve and explode it. Many times and exceptionally tiring thereafter." With a tank of 2 Kg (125-150 inflatables) he speeds up and could likewise arrange another one quicker. One more respondent discussions about his inflatable companions. First and foremost they would begin with one tank, yet that before long would become a few all at once. No one idea it was habit-forming in light of the fact that they didn't utilize consistently. "It was simply fun. Also, it makes young ladies insane and turned on. We put a great deal of gas in lodgings. I paid the daily pace of 120 euros. We snuck the tank into the rucksack. Both of us went in and afterward one returned to get two others" (Man, 21 years of age).

In any case, not every person responded in a casual way to nitrous oxide. "Nitrous oxide was a genuine publicity. Things began to go crazy as it was utilized in bigger gatherings. Feelings frequently ran high, there were contentions while others were stumbling on that gas. They saw things that were not there. You find that you like to be separated from everyone else or in a little gathering without interruption" (Lady, 27).

After the "trial stage", use is expanded in works in the "party stage". After a rich period, the first gathering gradually breaks down and psychologists to a little center of clients that continues onward and won't stop. Clients who in the end up in the pinnacle stage become progressively separated and "gorge" on their own something like three times each week on a few 2-Kg tanks per meeting, or one 2-Kg tank practically every day. The most extreme somebody utilized was around eight tanks in a day-long gorge. One loves huge inflatables (fine balls), while the other likes to breathe in more modest inflatables (one every moment). None of the youngsters talked with said they had a breaking point. Basically on the grounds that they rapidly lose count and keep on utilizing "by feeling". Some enter an immortal vacuum during their nitrous oxide gorge where hours and days appear to converge into one long outing. "You nod off with an inflatable in your mouth, awaken following 90 minutes, and happen with inflatables" (Man, 22 years of age).

At this stage, most didn't understand that wellbeing chances were expanding essentially. "I heard tales about individuals getting deadened, yet additionally saw that everybody around me continued to make it happen. In the event that they can deal with that much, then my body can deal with considerably more", flaunted one respondent (male, 20 years of age). The respondents gave different explanations behind changing to tricky use. A couple of respondents said that the indistinct universe of nitrous oxide gives impermanent help. At any rate, you don't need to contemplate your aggravation and issues that you can't tackle. One respondent (Man, 29 years of age) says he began utilizing more nitrous oxide a couple of years prior for more unwinding. Nonetheless, the hidden explanation was that he had a "burnout" because of a high responsibility and was stuck due to the struggles at home (actually resides with his folks). "At the point when I was worried, I would go outside to involve nitrous oxide as a flight. My head felt so full that it seemed like help from the get go." In any case, at one point he could never again switch appropriately between his work and his nitrous propensity around evening time. One respondent (ladies, 27 years of age) escalated nitrous oxide utilize following a horrendous mishap (scared and undermined by two obscure men). She felt troubled and began utilizing a great deal to mute her considerations and changed to tanks. She knew an adequate number of sellers. As she at this point not believed anybody, she began involving it consistently for quite some time; alone in the vehicle on the edges of Amsterdam with a 2-Kg tank that required her six hours. "For me it was eat, work, call the seller, and use it and rest. Consistently for a very long time." The sellers were content with her since she likewise presented different clients so she at times got a tank for nothing. Another respondent (Man, 26 years of age) was guileless about the lawbreaker twofold existence of his companions. At the point when the police looked for him, he crawled under a rock for a long time and wound up in a ratty universe of private gatherings, get-togethers, shisha parlors and transitory sanctuaries. He began utilizing nitrous oxide to an ever increasing extent, and in higher dosages to lessen the pressure that had emerged. There are additionally youngsters who steadily began utilizing nitrous oxide to an ever increasing extent. One respondent (Man, 19 years of age) worked in deals and thereafter went on a nitrous oxide visit with a couple of partners. He said: " We began with 2 Kg (75 inflatables each), yet that gradually expanded to 8-10 Kg. We happened until 3 a.m. - 4 a.m., when the tank was vacant. You are developing resistance, you know, which makes you need to utilize increasingly more each time." At the outset he generally utilized with companions on ends of the week however wound up alone, alongside his tank in his vehicle close by a parking garage. "I simply needed to space, so you can continue to thunder. You needed to remain in it. No, I had no restriction."

Because of expanding resistance (adjustment), the degree of the utilization of nitrous oxide can rapidly build, which can prompt tricky or unreasonable use. "The main inflatables consistently feel better; then the loathsomeness begins", one respondent said (Man, 21 years of age). At the point when the Netherlands went into "lockdown" because of Coronavirus, he began to "develop musicality" and he "shot" three 2-Kg tanks three times each week and in the middle between. A year prior, he was the jaunty kid who organized tanks, lodgings and young ladies anxious to set up a party. In any case, he changed character and began to show flighty way of behaving; immediately ended up being furious and had angry outbursts when young ladies needed to return home. "I was desolate, had exited school and the tank turned into my dearest companion. I rested in the vehicle in carports."

Unfavorable Wellbeing Impacts of Dangerous Use

The main indications of actual harm because of nitrous oxide use are shivering in your toes and feet, losing balance all the more rapidly and falls become more normal. Different side effects are vascular difficulties and infarcts, feeling swelled and sickened, acid reflux, major irritation, the upper arms and shoulders and one's actual strength can "totally" vanish in six months or less. Frostbite wounds have happened, in light of the fact that the tank becomes super cold during depleting, which isn't seen because of the sedative impact of nitrous oxide. A few clients get rankles in the mouth, and on the tongue, arms and legs. A portion of the injuries are exceptionally profound and recuperating is hazardous, requiring various medical procedures and bringing about scars with low quality. "It was as of now not simple to hold a pen. Composing turned out to be more troublesome. My words were likewise more terrible" (Lady, 27 years of age). The actual grievances are not extremely durable and (may some of the time) vanish. Numerous clients clearly don't yet understand the connection between their exorbitant use and expanding actual uneasiness, finishing them up in the peril zone. "My longing for nitrous oxide was more grounded than my psyche", said one respondent (Man, 19 years of age). Until he was unable to get up on the grounds that his legs were deadened. He was raced to emergency clinic by rescue vehicle. After a talk from the specialist and vitamin B12 infusions, he was in a good place again half a month after the fact. Once at home, he began utilizing once more and was readmitted following a couple of months. Because of their exorbitant use, a few respondents turned out to be (briefly) deadened in their legs, yet generally recuperated after concentrated treatment. One respondent (Man, 26 years of age) actually can't understand the reason why he didn't hear alerts when his neighbor wound up in a wheelchair.

Dangerous clients of nitrous oxide additionally revealed mental issues. The respondents revealed high pressure, squabbles and now and again savagery between clients or toward companions, accomplices and guardians. Weighty clients can become capricious and neurotic dreams can prompt fierce way of behaving. During our hands on work, we needed to painstakingly move toward the vehicles with clients in them, since they are in their self-made time container. An unpleasant unsettling influence can prompt forceful way of behaving. One respondent (Man, 29 years of age) felt he had become missing and retained in his self, subsequent to utilizing nitrous oxide. Weighty clients can abruptly become forceful he cautioned. "Never thump on a vehicle window where somebody is separating a tank, since you can cause problems."

Grievances detailed by respondents during their gorge of many inflatables at a time and often in excess of a thousand seven days are emotional episodes, mental breakdowns, neurosis and once in a while self-destructive considerations. Weighty nitrous oxide use supports gloomy feelings: high portions of nitrous oxide can prompt dreams, fantasies and a sensation of depersonalization. "You will converse with your tank and see things that aren't there" one respondent (Man, 29 years of age) told. He turned out to be neurotic to such an extent that he needed to drive away to escape the underhanded spirits. At some other point, he thought the young lady, with whom he frequently utilized nitrous oxide, was attempting to trap him. One respondent (Man, 21 years of age) said that he makes things greater in his mind. At the point when he utilizes alone in the vehicle, he hears various voices that can very bother. He got terrified and distrustful that somebody planned to hurt him. Once he went nuts and put a weapon to his sanctuary. "In the space, you see odd things. I saw individuals go to dark smoke. In the event that you are a devotee, you get restless when Satan camouflages himself in hallucinations" (Man, 26 years of age). Flashbacks likewise happen. One respondent (Lady, 27 years of age) depicted remembering awful recollections of her dad in adolescence; nitrous oxide makes dreams that take you to an obscure hidden world. One more respondent got into a confidence and character emergency, on the grounds that nitrous oxide turned his reasoning and conviction world tops curvy. He looked for help from a sort of imam, who encouraged him to quit utilizing nitrous oxide; you will then naturally get back to the unadulterated way. "As a

Muslim you must areas of strength for be you realize that you are committing a transgression assuming that you use drugs or nitrous oxide. Numerous young men begin to contemplate their convictions when they are impaired and get into struggle with themselves. That is hard to make sense of. It's exceptionally confounding and you can't actually converse with anybody about it. You should address it yourself, yet you don't have the foggiest idea how. That makes a ton of additional strain" (Man, 26 years of age).

Social and Monetary Issues

The first joy of sporting nitrous oxide may continuously form into constant utilize that is connected to physical, mental and social grumblings. During the meeting, a few respondents acknowledged interestingly that they might have infrequently been maniacal or had encountered pipedreams. The weighty clients bit by bit disengage themselves, as a result of contentions in the bigger gathering. A model is in the story that weighty clients frequently end up in a vehicle some place in a neglected spot, alongside his tank, a sack of inflatables and a telephone to call his seller when the tank is practically unfilled. "One needs music, the other doesn't; he needs to hear this, the other that once more. Discussions at times upset you. Everybody needs the best circumstance for themselves. Furthermore, that makes strain" (Man, 19 years of age). Clients fall into social separation: exited from school, got terminated and blew up with that last cherished one who thinks often about you. "You lose everything, your better half, your companions, school, and I was removed from home. You live in an air pocket. Everything revolves around inflatables" (Man, 21 years of age). Obligation collection is likewise an issue. You begin purchasing tanks on layaway from sellers who lash out on the off chance that you don't pay on time, yet you frantically need another tank. "While I was utilizing, Nitrous was the main thing I could imagine. I continued to guarantee my vendor that I would get him the cash rapidly (1500-euro obligation), in any event, when I didn't have it any longer. I continued rationalizing and abusing his trust. The cash will come tomorrow! I got back on layaway for 10 Kg. He continued to give it to me and I continued deferring paying" (Man, 19 years of age). His vendor got tired of his accounts and begun compromising him, however his sister, to whom he previously owed EUR 11,000, saved him that evening just under the wire.

Restrictions on Admittance to Treatment

Weighty clients generally deny the issues related with risky nitrous oxide use by persevering in their conviction that nitrous oxide is innocuous. What's more, they barely seem to talk about such issues with others, and at first minimize their utilization, dangers and individual issues. Thusly, their interest for help is insignificant in light of the fact that the issues are deficiently perceived by their immediate climate. It was at that point obvious that substance use, and all the more explicitly nitrous oxide use, are no subjects about which youngsters in the parent culture can't straightforwardly trade thoughts. Most respondents get little assistance and should tackle their nitrous oxide issues themselves. A few respondents allude to their way of life where it is many times about pride and honor and that you would rather not harm your standing. To that end clients like to keep those considerations (issues) to themselves. Some thusly discuss a "culture of quietness" in which you keep your mouth shut about others. In road culture, ending the quietness to the specialists is frequently condemned as "squealing". Numerous respondents said that they could do without to converse with their folks about their sentiments, feelings, and fears, regardless of whether they would comprehend. A vibe that their folks' capacity to comprehend is restricted so it would just make additional problem. They are routinely told from home "not to wander off-track". One respondent (Man, 19 years of age) said that his mom told him not to stow away assuming he planned to give things a shot; he could constantly converse with her about it. "But I found it hard to discuss nitrous oxide. I was additionally embarrassed about myself and felt that I was not prepared for help." Another respondent (Lady, 19 years of age) said that she doesn't discuss it at home, since she fears frustrating her folks. "My folks think I'm a youngster wonder. And afterward I will let you know that I do expands consistently? Precisely what my dad generally cautioned me against. I don't tell companions. They have a bias that I am staying here." Another respondent (Man, 19 years of age) additionally feels remorseful toward his folks now that he is in Reade restoration community for treatment. He wouldn't even play with the possibility of confronting them and is glad that his more seasoned sibling is a middle person. He feels crushed for harming their pride for him. He feels extremely remorseful about that and feels like he has fizzled.

A few respondents said that moms, sisters or aunties frequently show the most sympathy and proposition the arrangement; fathers like to be "kept unaware of everything going on" however much as could reasonably be expected. They reached the specialist or therapist, e.g., for the reference. It is frequently challenging for young men to discuss their sentiments with other young men. They are in reality as we know it where everything revolves around boasting, achievement, sturdiness, looking great, dazzling young ladies, showing that you have balls. Beside the manly reason, don't irritate others with "your poop" since they are many times wrecked themselves. " You have your pride. You shut up, in light of the fact that all of a sudden, tattle is happening around that you have issues" (Man, 26 years of age). For sure, Moroccan young men are hesitant to partake in bunch treatment presented by habit care, where they should discuss their feelings; they are not by any stretch of the imagination used to talking transparently about their concerns, so they frequently quit. Then again, a few respondents have been moved toward by concerned companions about their super nitrous oxide use; a few even many times. Nonetheless, because of expanding disconnection, the rest of the world is getting progressively less mindful of it. It is critical that a few respondents can examine their concern with an obscure or "safe" individual who is figuring out, not moralistic and ignorant about their friend network. Someone who isn't threating and doesn't think you are a terrible Muslim.

Advising by Muslim Pastorate and Experts

All respondents said they couldn't or reluctant to impart their concerns to their folks. They additionally didn't have any desire to annoy their companions, since they were battling with similar issues. The refusal of practically all respondents to counsel an expert (youth or social specialist in the field) or social laborer is roused by pride, disgrace or forswearing of the issue. Besides, they don't have any idea how help is coordinated and are once in a while terrified of winding up "in a framework". So, most hazardous clients continue to tangle on and said that they don't have a decent connection with experts or don't think that they are trustworthy, in light of the fact that they don't comprehend the Moroccan culture well.

The guide to the respondents seems to follow two tracks: first the Moroccan methodology (basically according to the honest perspective) trailed by help in light of the Dutch methodology (brain science, clinical). As per the exhortation of guardians, companions or relatives, a Moroccan otherworldly guide or care supplier is first reached, with whom mental issues connected with the utilization of nitrous oxide can be examined. One respondent (Man, 21 years of age) a the talked about an imam sections of Satan from the Blessed Quran to project out Satan. Another respondent (Man, 29 years of age) first went to Morocco for a nitrous oxide detox to find "inward harmony". After his return, notwithstanding, he immediately fell once more into weighty use, after which he was owned up to Reade for a spinal string injury.

One respondent (Man, 29 years of age) first went to Morocco for help and afterward looked for help in Amsterdam. "They (the jellied compulsion office) truly helped me and gave me an understanding into how it functions for me when I need nitrous oxide. It assisted me with getting to realize my conduct better." He said that this information additionally assists him have better discussions with companions and to attempt to help them. "I let them know that they don't need to be so scared of Dutch guide, since it helped me a great deal. I went to Morocco for an Islamic fix. Many refrains from the Heavenly Quran are then perused to remove the shaytaan (Satan). I felt that I was settling once more. I could never have done that here. You fail to remember what you're doing here and break your day to day schedules" (Man, 29 years of age).

Notwithstanding the "good times" side about nitrous oxide via virtual entertainment [2], there are now video blogs on YouTube in which imams express their interests about nitrous oxide. It is thusly worth thinking about utilizing forces to be reckoned with (good examples) in crusades, focused on the dangers and treatment of weighty nitrous oxide use.

Conversation

The quantity of nitrous oxide related wellbeing episodes has consistently arisen in the beyond three years and prompted expanding worry at recovery focuses, the crisis division and fixation care in Amsterdam. Notwithstanding the arising unfavorable wellbeing impacts, a consistently developing number of car crashes, where the driver was affected by nitrous oxide, have been accounted for. A developing gathering of mostly youthful transients (a couple dozen every year), specifically Moroccan-Dutch youth, have created extreme utilization of nitrous oxide. Consequently, the city board intends to go to additional lengths (crusade online powerhouses, outreach work) among gatherings of continuous (dangerous) clients who know nothing about the dangers of nitrous oxide.

Nitrous Oxide Use in an Untouchable Culture

The main inquiry of the request was about the contentions why subjects wished to abstain from nitrous oxide use. All clients referenced the extraordinary untouchable on liquor and substance use in their religion and parent culture. Guardians frequently have practically zero involvement in substance use and have subsequently a restricted casing of reference. Drugs are haram (precluded) and guardians maintain that their kids should feel the same way. The ongoing age of youngsters somewhat gets this message (blocking factor), however there is likewise a significant gathering that begins to try in the juvenile stage since they come to settings (going out, hanging out, adolescent confinement, excursion, and so forth.), where the untouchable on substance use is pretty much overlooked or purposely abused. Be that as it may, what thought processes do youngsters have for encountering nitrous oxide in an untouchable culture? Youngsters who are in this course of assimilation feel a specific pressure on the grounds that the infringement of rules and the disinhibitory conduct are in conflict with the rules of the confidence that opposes or denies the utilization of intoxicants. This restraint worldview, where there is by all accounts no center way (self-guideline) between all out forbearance or fixation, is suggestive of the senseless hysteria encompassing youthful medication clients in frequently stringently strict Dutch fishing towns.

With the exception of a little gathering of hazardous clients (principally Moroccan and Turkish youth), most sporting nitrous oxide clients don't experience drug related issues. Drug clients may, notwithstanding, experience drug related issues, in the event that set and setting are in misbalance. The set and setting are made sense of in the model of Finberg [54]. As per this model (1) segment and social-monetary qualities of the client, the thought processes, discernment, past involvement in different medications and the individual mentality towards the substance ("the set") and (2) the social and actual climate wherein drug use happens ("the setting") are definitive for the positive or negative insight of a substance. Becker [55] recently contended that controlled medication use is the consequence of a growing experience in the friend bunch. At long last, it might have been pertinent for the particular gathering explored here, that medication use can likewise be a departure from the regular hackneyed daily practice or a response to an instable and quickly impacting world in which without adequate social control, the desire extravagantly and kicks is amplified.

The truth of the matter is that youngsters experience an inward struggle and, out of a specific regard for their folks, begin to feel more remorseful. Accordingly, youngsters exploring different avenues regarding drugs like to do as such beyond their neighborhood to keep away from tattle and social control. They should continually think of reasons and deceives to cover the utilization of liquor, pot or different substances (smell, conduct, being impaired, and so forth.). Accordingly, nitrous oxide gives an optimal vindication: the air is unscented, and the impact isn't conspicuous to the rest of the world and guardians and isn't noticeable in the way of behaving. Some even think that since it is air, that the substance isn't held in the body.

Nitrous oxide use was worked with, particularly among youngsters, by its low cost, obvious security, simple access and legitimate status. The epicurean clasp culture, where celebrating young people use in a lighthearted way, has likewise added to the ubiquity. The coming of huge kilo tanks, given by aggressive day in and day out conveyance administrations, has been an emotional major advantage. From that second on, because of more straightforward tapping of the gas, the quickly expanding adjustment, and the likelihood to breathe in nitrous oxide constant, continued dosing appears to be limitless. An extensive gathering of clueless clients slowly breathe in themselves longer and more profound into an obscure world without a base, roof, and viewpoint. Some of them progressively become mixed up in entrancingly redundant and durable nitrous oxide meetings beginning from one time per week, to a couple of times each week to here and there each day. Contrasted with different substances, nitrous oxide is different in that it very well may be utilized for quite a long time and in some cases even days (gorge) and the client doesn't know when he/she needs to stop.

Low Information and Hazard Insight

The second inquiry of the examination alluded to the gamble impression of (regular) nitrous oxide use and how much this impacted their degree of purpose. At first, the respondents didn't group nitrous oxide as a risky substance in light of its "guiltless" nature, strikingly on the grounds that it was not habit-forming, as affirmed by specialists. Furthermore, nitrous oxide is offered all over the place. Additionally, this gathering of substance clients feels little need to illuminate themselves and to share their insight about the impacts, doses and potential wellbeing gambles. Particularly youngsters with a scholarly handicap experience troubles in understanding the data about the dangers of nitrous oxide as dispersed by drug counteraction associations. Conversely, clasps of specialists encompassed by hip-influencing young ladies with inflatables and cool folks who give additional choke with inflatables in the driver's seat are frequently shared by (road) young people. In that type, recordings of fender benders are generally seen, shared and remarked on. Conversations about nitrous oxide on the Web among great and miscreants are likewise exceptionally famous. The upsides of road culture now and again reverberate in the way of behaving encompassing inflatable use. You would rather not perform more terrible than others and you outperform the others with considerably more inflatables. In that capacity, the dangers are searched out as opposed to kept away from. Besides, youngsters (i.e., the respondents talked with) are guileless and uninformed about psychoactive substances, since they have little involvement in them themselves and have no companions who have such insight and information. Evidently, without the consciousness of wellbeing takes a chance with an automatic system is generally deficient. It might happen that somebody, as a decent Muslim, has never at any point smoked tobacco or tipsy liquor, yet goes totally off course on nitrous oxide in a brief time frame.

Treatment Interest

The risky clients and previous clients who were consulted begun utilizing nitrous oxide more regularly and in progressively higher portions in light of multiple factors. They can be generally defined into those with a connection to road culture and (at times) with contacts in youth and social work in the field, and those with no or powerless binds with road culture and have entered the work market subsequent to having completed their schooling (frequently halfway professional training). They submerged themselves in the celebrations, couldn't stay aware of the time, or turned out to be unfastened (some of the time out of fatigue). Some experienced mental pressure (jobless or high work pressure and the desire to perform) or experienced an unsound home circumstance, an absence of acknowledgment and appreciation, or Post Horrible Pressure Issue (PTSD).

Nitrous oxide gave impermanent alleviation to everybody, with the outcome that the issues accepted turned out to be more awful as they utilized more nitrous oxide. In time, this prompted different (serious) actual objections, mental issues and social avoidance due to exorbitant use. Respondents (particularly in their maltreatment stage) experienced numerous hindrances to discuss individual contemplations that irritation or disappoint them as well as issues that emerge because of misuse. They will generally minimize their predicament and could do without to communicate their concerns: not to their folks, ideally not to companions, and absolutely not to their "road companions". Frequently youngsters say that their pride and honor are in question and they like to hush up about their concerns. The feeling of disappointment, including such somebody's reality isn't satisfying their folks' assumptions, is far and wide.

The constant exchanging between various universes (home, school and friend network) takes a great deal of energy. Youngsters frequently find it hard to discuss sentiments and feelings. The pressure of character, execution and social control between their own local area and Dutch society is additionally reflected in the ongoing outcomes. During the time of their weighty use, the respondents stayed away from (looking for) help, or potentially rejected that they were experiencing (serious) close to home issues. With regards to dangerous nitrous oxide use (in an untouchable culture), it is possible that some — on the power of their current circumstance (counting guardians, companions) — first looked for shelter with an imam or customary healer. Plus, youngsters say that they don't have adequate trust in help by local Dutch clinical guardians or doubt their assistance. Also, they are new to them or don't have the foggiest idea how to reach them.

Restrictions of the Review

Mostly because of troublesome admittance to tricky nitrous oxide clients beyond institutional settings and the weighty obstruction by sensations of disgrace among Moroccan young people who utilize nitrous oxide in a hazardous manner, the example may not be completely delegate and hence doesn't mirror a genuinely irregular example. All subjects were enlisted from the Dutch-Moroccan people group, suggesting that the outcomes are not delegate for Dutch society.

Epilog

Until this point, essentially no exploration has been led into the advancement of hazardous nitrous oxide use. The meetings with Moroccan-Dutch youths yielded an abundance of data about their current circumstance (counting home, school, companions, extra energy), their perspectives on liquor and medication use as a general rule, and nitrous oxide use specifically, their drives to utilize increasingly more nitrous oxide and how their current circumstance approaches substance use in the strict no culture.

As a team with Reade, Jellied and the young work in Amsterdam, New-West, we had the one of a kind chance to talk with this gathering of youngsters (with their consent) top to bottom. Their own accounts gave a more honed and more nuanced image of the basic social and social components connected with (hazardous) drug use in Moroccan-Dutch youth culture, including their treatment interest. The substance of the meetings will be utilized to calibrate a designated decrease technique for risky nitrous oxide use in this gathering. Probably, the ongoing outcomes likewise give an opening to those (guardians, companions, experts, and so forth.) who are gone up against with such dangerous clients. Any individual who thinks for even a moment to humanely go into a discussion with youngsters will ideally acquire a superior comprehension concerning why a few clients actually see their nitrous oxide tank as their as it were "companion".

Nitrous oxide-based methods versus nitrous oxide-free strategies for general sedation

Nitrous oxide has been utilized for north of 160 years for the acceptance and upkeep of general sedation. It has been utilized as a sole specialist yet is most frequently utilized as a feature of a strategy utilizing other sedative gases, intravenous specialists, or both. Its low tissue solvency (and consequently quick energy), minimal expense, and low pace of cardiorespiratory confusions have made nitrous oxide by a long shot the most usually utilized general sedative. The gathering proof with respect to unfriendly impacts of nitrous oxide organization has driven numerous anesthetists to scrutinize it's proceeded with routine use in an assortment of working room settings. Unfriendly occasions might result from both the natural activities of nitrous oxide and the way that to convey a compelling portion, nitrous oxide, which is a moderately powerless sedative specialist, should be given in high fixations that limit oxygen conveyance (for instance, a typical blend is 30% oxygen with 70% nitrous oxide). As well as the gamble of low blood oxygen levels, concerns have likewise been raised with respect to the gamble of giving and taking the resistant framework, disabled comprehension, postoperative cardiovascular confusions, and entrails obstacle from expansion, and conceivable respiratory split the difference.

We included randomized controlled preliminaries (RCTs) looking at general sedation where nitrous oxide was important for the sedative procedure utilized for the enlistment or support of general sedation (or both) with any broad sedation utilizing an unpredictable sedative or propofol-based upkeep of sedation however no nitrous oxide for grown-ups going through a medical procedure. Our essential result was in hospital case casualty rate. Optional results were inconveniences and length of stay.

Information assortment and examination

Two survey creators autonomously evaluated preliminary quality and removed the result information. We utilized meta-analysis for information union. Heterogeneity was inspected with the Chi^2 test and by ascertaining the I^2 measurement. We utilized a fixed-effect model on the off chance that the proportion of irregularity was low for all correlations (I^2 measurement < half); in any case we utilized a random-effects model for measures with high irregularity. We attempted subgroup investigations to investigate irregularity and awareness examinations to assess whether the outcomes were powerful. We surveyed the nature of proof of the principal results utilizing the Reviewing of Suggestions, Appraisal, Advancement and Assessment (GRADE) framework.

Primary outcomes

We included 35 preliminaries (13,872 grown-up members). Seven included examinations were at generally safe of inclination. We recognized eight investigations as anticipating grouping since we were unable to acquire the full texts, and had lacking data to incorporate or bar them. We included information from 24 preliminaries for quantitative amalgamation. The consequences of meta-analyses showed that nitrous oxide-based strategies expanded the frequency of aspiratory atelectasis (chances proportion (OR) 1.57, 95% certainty span (CI) 1.18 to 2.10, P = 0.002), yet no affected the in hospital case casualty rate, the occurrence of pneumonia, myocardial localized necrosis, stroke, extreme queasiness and retching, venous thromboembolism, wound contamination, or the length of clinic stay. The responsiveness examinations proposed that the consequences of the meta-analyses were all hearty aside from the results of pneumonia, and extreme sickness and spewing. Two preliminaries announced length of emergency unit stay however the information were slanted so were not pooled. The two preliminaries announced that nitrous oxide-based procedures no affected the length of ICU stay. We appraised the nature of proof for two results (pneumonic atelectasis, myocardial localized necrosis) as high, four results (in hospital case casualty rate, stroke, venous thromboembolism, length of medical clinic stay) as moderate, and three (pneumonia, serious sickness and heaving, wound disease rate) as low.

Creators' decisions

Given the proof from this Cochrane survey, the aversion of nitrous oxide might be sensible in members with pre-existing poor aspiratory capability or at high gamble of postoperative sickness and heaving. Since there are eight examinations anticipating characterization, choice predisposition might exist in our precise survey.

Nitrous oxide is a sedative gas which has been utilized for over 160 years for instigating sedation and keeping patients anesthetized all through an activity. It is otherwise called 'giggling gas'. It is a boring non-flammable gas with a lovely, faint sweet smell and taste. Its minimal expense and low poisonousness have made nitrous oxide by a wide margin the most regularly utilized general sedative. Nonetheless, a few examinations have detailed that adding nitrous oxide might prompt unsafe impacts. This has driven numerous anesthetists to scrutinize it's proceeded with routine use in an assortment of working room settings.

Nitrous oxide, otherwise called giggling gas, is a drab non-flammable gas with a charming, faintly sweet smell and taste. The gas has been in need for over 160 years for the enlistment and upkeep of general sedation. It has been utilized as a sole specialist yet is most frequently utilized as a feature of a strategy utilizing other sedative gases, intravenous specialists, or both. Its low tissue solvency (and consequently quick energy), minimal expense, and low pace of cardiorespiratory confusions have made nitrous oxide by a long shot the most usually utilized general sedative. Around the world, it is given to more than one billion careful patients yearly (Fleischmann 2005).

The gathering proof in regards to unfavorable impacts of nitrous oxide organization has driven numerous anesthetists to scrutinize it's proceeded with routine use in an assortment of working room settings. Unfriendly occasions might result from both the natural activities of nitrous oxide and the way that to convey a compelling portion, nitrous oxide, which is a moderately powerless sedative specialist, should be given in high fixations that limit oxygen conveyance (for instance, a typical blend is 30% oxygen with 70% nitrous oxide).

The burdens of nitrous oxide have been accounted for. Concerns have been raised in regards to the gamble of giving and taking the safe framework (Par brook 1967), low blood oxygen levels (Cheney 2007), debilitated discernment (mental capacity) (Culley 2007; Linde 1969), postoperative cardiovascular inconveniences (Myles 2008b), as well as inside impediment from widening and conceivable respiratory split the difference (Eger 1965). Moreover, nitrous oxide might build the gamble of creating mind harm from decreased cerebral blood stream (Lehmberg 2008; Pasternak 2009). At last, nitrous oxide is a demonstrated gamble factor for queasiness and spewing (Apfel 2004).

Depiction of the mediation

As a powerless sedative, nitrous oxide is for the most part not utilized alone in everyday sedation. In spite of the fact that there is extensive variety in how this medication is utilized, an ordinary situation would be the upkeep of careful sedation, for anything that period expected, by the organization of 69% nitrous oxide, 29% oxygen, and 2% of a strong unpredictable sedative specialist, for example, sevoflurane. On the other hand, an intravenous medication could be persistently mixed while the patient inhales 70% nitrous oxide and 30% oxygen. The impact of nitrous oxide is to decrease the portion of either an unpredictable or intravenous sedative that is expected to keep a proper degree of sedation.

How the intercession could function

Similarly as with other vaporous sedative specialists, the specific instrument of activity of nitrous oxide isn't totally perceived. Hypotheses incorporate enmity at both the N-methyl-D-aspartate (NMDA) excitatory receptors and focal nicotinic receptors; what's more, a comparable inhibitory impact at the two-pore K+ channel TWIK-related potassium channel-1 (TREK-1), a potassium direct engaged with polymodal torment discernment, to show pain relieving, anxiolytic, and amnesic properties (Gruss 2004; Jevtović-Todorović 1998; Yama Kura 2000).

As proposed above, nitrous oxide is in many cases utilized as one part of a fair sedative methodology. This enjoys a few potential benefits remembering a decrease for the prerequisites for different specialists, and thusly a diminished rate and seriousness of any unfriendly impacts of those specialists, a quick beginning of sedative impact, and a more fast recuperation of cognizance once the sedation is ended (Becker 2008). These benefits should be adjusted against the expected drawbacks of nitrous oxide. Unthinkingly, a considerable lot of the unfriendly impacts of nitrous oxide are credited to the inactivation of the coalman type of vitamin B12, by oxidation, in this manner restraining the activity of methionine synthase, folate digestion, and deoxyribonucleic corrosive combination. These are significant for protein creation and DNA union (Guirguis 1990; Perry 1983; Rowland 1995). Additionally, nitrous oxide pushes down a white cells' capacity to answer different improvements and decreases the development of other white cell components (mononucleocytes) (Kripke 1987).

Why doing this review is significant

As nitrous oxide organization brings the two benefits and weaknesses, an orderly survey will help the singular anesthetist in settling on the most proper decision of sedative strategy on a singular patient premise. The equilibrium of hazard versus benefit is probably going to rely upon many variables. The point of this Cochrane audit was to quantitatively assess assuming nitrous oxide was liable for clinically huge unfavorable occasions following general sedation that could be securely kept away from by the utilization of elective specialists. This might broadly affect the direct of general sedation.

Two survey writers (RS, WQJ) created and utilized a normalized information extraction structure as per the Cochrane Handbook for Efficient Surveys of Intercessions (Higgins 2011). Two audit creators (RS, XFL) autonomously registered and entered information with Reedman 5.3 for factual examination.

Determination of studies one audit writer (WQJ) checked the titles and modified works of articles recovered by the inquiry and eliminated those that didn't meet our consideration standards. Three survey creators (JHT, WQJ, and RS) recovered the full text of all possibly qualified examinations. Two survey writers (RS, WQJ) freely analyzed the full text articles for consistence with the consideration standards and chose reads up qualified for incorporation in the audit. We settled any conflict as to concentrate on qualification by conversation with a third survey creator (KHY).

Information extraction and the board

We separated information from qualified investigations utilizing an information structure we had planned and pilot-tested (Supplement 5). At the point when a concentrate either covered or was a copy of another review, WQ Jia and P Zhang reached the review creators for explanation and, whenever affirmed, involved the distribution with the more itemized information for this deliberate survey and consolidated the extra information. Two survey creators (RS, PZ) reached the first review creators for extra information for included results that were not distributed in the review. Two survey creators (WQJ,

RS) freely separated the information and settled any conflict by counseling a third survey creator (KHY).

We extricated the accompanying data:

Concentrate on plan (RCT).

Members (number, age, orientation, American Culture of Anesthesiologists (ASA) actual status grouping, infection, sort of a medical procedure).

Intercession (convergence of nitrous oxide, blended breathed in sedative, centralization of oxygen, span of breathed in nitrous oxide).

Quality evaluation (grouping age, portion covering, blinding, fragmented result information, different issues).

Result (essential and auxiliary results, strategies used to survey results, season of follow-up).

Evaluation of chance of predisposition in included examinations Two survey creators (RS, BM) freely surveyed the nature of the investigations by building a 'Hazard of inclination's table for each study which included succession age, designation camouflage, blinding, deficient result information, specific revealing, and other predisposition (Higgins 2011). Any conflicts were settled by conversation between the two audit creators.

We evaluated the quality variables of each concentrate independently. These were named either 'low', 'high', or 'hazy' chance of inclination.

Proportions of treatment impact considering dichotomous factors, we communicated the distinction in the quantity of occasions in the nitrous oxide-based bunch and the nitrous oxide-free bunch as a chances proportion (OR) for entanglements and Pete chances proportion (Pete OR) for the in hospital case casualty rate. For length of stay, we just pooled the information communicated as mean and standard deviation (SD). The impact size for length of stay was the mean distinction (MD). We introduced 95% certainty stretches (CIs) for all results.

Unit of investigation issues non-standard plan RCTs can introduce measurable issues. While we didn't expect to incorporate hybrid or bunch randomized plans in this Cochrane survey, we expected different mediation gatherings. We took care to stay away from 'unit of investigation's blunders while breaking down these kinds of preliminaries (Higgins 2011).

Managing missing information in case of missing information, two survey creators (WQJ, RS) attempted to contact the creators of the first examinations to acquire the vital data. Two survey creators (XFL, RS) dissected the information on an intention-to-treat (ITT) premise beyond what many would consider possible.

Evaluation of heterogeneity

We thought about whether the clinical and systemic qualities of the included investigations were adequately comparable for meta-analysis to give a significant outline. Measurably, we analyzed heterogeneity with the Chi^2 test and by ascertaining the I^2 measurement. We believed heterogeneity to be significant when the I^2 measurement > half and painstakingly thought to be the information prior to detailing any pooled results (Higgins 2002). In the event that significant heterogeneity was distinguished, we investigated potential clarifications in subgroup examinations.

Evaluation of detailing predispositions

We directed an extensive quest for qualified investigations. On the off chance that there were at least 10 examinations in an investigation, we utilized a pipe plot to investigate the chance of distribution predisposition and other detailing predispositions. In the examinations for dichotomous results we additionally evaluated distribution predisposition measurably with the utilization of Egger's test (Egger 1997) performed with Stata 11.0. We put together proof of imbalance with respect to $P < 0.05$.

Information blend

We utilized meta-analysis for information union. We utilized a fixed-effect model on the off chance that the proportion of irregularity was low for all correlations (I^2 measurement < half); in any case we utilized a random-effects model for measures with high irregularity. Where we didn't lead meta-analysis, we depicted the discoveries of the included investigations subjectively.

We remembered the accompanying results for the 'Rundown of discoveries' tables:

In hospital case casualty rate.

Pneumonia.

Aspiratory atelectasis.

Myocardial localized necrosis.

Stroke.

Serious queasiness and spewing.

Length of emergency clinic stay.

Venous thromboembolism.

Wound contamination rate.

We appraised the nature of proof for every result keeping the rules of Reviewing of Suggestions, Appraisal, Advancement and Assessment (GRADE) approach (Schumann 2009) and in view of the accompanying five downsize factors: hazard of predisposition, irregularity, aberrance, imprecision, and distribution inclination. For each downsize factor, a judgment of 'no', 'serious (minimize the nature of proof by one level)', or 'intense (downsize the nature of proof by two levels)' was doled out. At the earliest reference point, we grouped every one of the results as at 'top notch' of course, and in the wake of rating, every result could get a grade of either 'high', 'moderate', 'low', or 'extremely bad' quality.

Subgroup examination and examination of heterogeneity
We embraced subgroup examinations as follows, as expressed in the Cochrane convention (Yang 2011):

Kind of medical procedure (day-case techniques/assessments versus intra-abdominal medical procedure versus neurosurgery versus vascular medical procedure versus ophthalmic medical procedure versus bosom a medical procedure).

Various centralizations of breathed in nitrous oxide (high fixation [higher than 50%] versus low focus [equal to or lower than 50%]).

Different mediation in the nitrous oxide-free bunch (propofol-based support of sedation versus unpredictable an aesthetic-based upkeep of sedation).

Responsiveness investigation To assess whether the consequences of the methodical audit were powerful, we led awareness examinations in view of the strategic quality (top notch versus bad quality) and the rates of withdrawals (above 10% versus underneath 10%) of the included RCTs.

We incorporated a sum of 35 preliminaries; seven of which were of okay of predisposition (Accad 2004; Arellano

2000; Mystery II preliminary 2014; Conundrum preliminary 2007; Fleischmann 2005; Lee 2005; Leung 2006). The meta-analyses uncovered that nitrous oxide-based procedures, contrasted and nitrous oxide-free strategies, expanded the frequency of aspiratory atelectasis however showed no distinction in the in hospital case casualty rate, the occurrence of pneumonia, myocardial localized necrosis, stroke, serious sickness and regurgitating, venous thromboembolism, wound disease, or the length of emergency clinic stay. Contrasted and nitrous oxide-free strategies, high-concentration nitrous oxide-based procedures expanded the rate of pneumonic atelectasis. Contrasted and either propofol-based or unpredictable an aesthetic-based sedation, nitrous oxide-based strategies meaningfully affected the in hospital case casualty rate, entanglements, or length of stay. The responsiveness investigations proposed that the consequences of meta-analyses were all vigorous aside from the results of pneumonia and serious queasiness and retching.

By and large culmination and appropriateness of proof

We included 13,872 grown-up members, who were of various ASA status going through various medical procedures. We contrasted various centralizations of nitrous oxide and nitrous oxide-free sedation, and furthermore contrasted nitrous oxide-based sedation and either propofol-based upkeep of sedation or unpredictable an aesthetic-based support of sedation. We focused harder on endpoints and patient-important results in resolving the inquiry with regards to whether nitrous oxide was answerable for clinically critical antagonistic occasions following general sedation. The meta-analyses results recommend that nitrous oxide brings about additional difficulties. Since the utilization of nitrous oxide in patients going through a medical procedure remains near-routine (de Violoncellos 2013), this methodical survey might broadly affect the direct of general sedation.

Nature of the proof

We included 35 RCTs, of which just 16 preliminaries portrayed the techniques for randomization and just 12 hid the distribution arrangement. As to, eight preliminaries detailed they dazed members and work force, while 25 preliminaries announced they dazed the result assessors.

Just seven of the 35 included preliminaries were at okay of inclination.

We recognized significant heterogeneity in the results of extreme queasiness and retching, wound contamination rate, and medical clinic stay, so we minimized the nature of proof for irregularity.

As the 95% CIs of ORs were wide for the results of in hospital case casualty rate, pneumonia, stroke, venous thromboembolism, and wound contamination rate, we downsized the nature of proof for these results because of imprecision.

At last, the nature of the proof for two results (pneumonic atelectasis, myocardial localized necrosis) was appraised as high, four results (in hospital case casualty rate, stroke, venous thromboembolism, and length of clinic stay) as moderate, and three (pneumonia, serious sickness and retching, wound contamination rate) as low; see Table 1 and Table 2.

Expected predispositions in the audit cycle

We led this Cochrane audit keeping the rules suggested in the Cochrane Handbook for Orderly Surveys of Mediations

(Higgins 2011) to limit predisposition. Notwithstanding, there are two issues that ought to be of concern. We, right off the bat, couldn't get the full texts of eight distributions through either our college library, the Danish Public Library, or Cochrane Sedation, Basic or Crisis Care Gathering individuals, so we might have missed likely qualified examinations. Consequently determination predisposition might exist in our precise audit. Also, significant heterogeneity was found in the result 'wound contamination rate', which was not made sense of by either subgroup examinations or awareness investigations. The heterogeneity appeared to be peculiar, and we pooled the information utilizing a random-effects model, which downsized our trust in this outcome.

Arrangements and conflicts with different examinations or surveys

In this Cochrane survey we contrasted nitrous oxide-based procedures and nitrous oxide-free methods on grown-up careful members, to decide if nitrous oxide was answerable for clinically critical unfriendly occasions following general sedation and whether nitrous oxide could be kept away from. There are likewise three precise surveys contrasting general sedation methods and or without nitrous oxide yet they center on postoperative sickness and spewing and intraoperative mindfulness. Two of these precise audits were distributed in 1996 (Divatia 1996; Tramèr 1996). Tramèr 1996 dissected the information on 2,478 members from 24 investigations and reasoned that precluding nitrous oxide from general sedatives altogether diminished the rate of postoperative regurgitating for patients at high gamble of spewing preoperatively, however affected the frequency of queasiness. They likewise found that discarding nitrous oxide expanded the gamble of intraoperative mindfulness. Divatia 1996 included 26 preliminaries and detailed that oversight of nitrous oxide decreased the chances of postoperative queasiness and regurgitating by 37%, a decrease in hazard of 28%. Fernández-Guisasola 2010 is another deliberate survey, and in contrast to the previous precise audits, Fernández-Guisasola 2010 barred pediatric reports. The creators included 30 examinations with 4598 grown-up members, and reasoned that keeping away from nitrous oxide lessens the gamble of postoperative queasiness and regurgitating, particularly in ladies, however the general effect was unobtrusive. In this Cochrane survey we additionally assessed the impacts of nitrous oxide on postoperative queasiness and spewing. In any case, we zeroed in on the frequency of extreme queasiness and spewing. We found that staying away from nitrous oxide might no affect the occurrence of extreme queasiness and regurgitating, yet the responsiveness examination proposed that the outcome was not vigorous. Imberger 2014 led an orderly survey with meta-analysis and preliminary successive examination, zeroing in on the impacts of nitrous oxide on mortality and cardiovascular grimness. The creators broke down the information of 13 preliminaries and found that nitrous oxide didn't influence either present moment (in the span of 30 days after activity) or long haul (beginning from 30 days after activity) mortality. Nonetheless, preliminary successive investigation showed that the information were unreasonably inadequate to make any ends. They didn't perform meta-analysis for cardiovascular entanglements (for example stroke, myocardial infarct, pneumonic embolus, heart failure) because of lacking information. Predictable with Limburger 2014, we additionally found that nitrous oxide-based sedation came about in comparative in hospital mortality contrasted and nitrous oxide-free sedation. Additionally, we pooled the information of cardiovascular confusions (for example myocardial dead tissue). The outcomes showed no tremendous distinction in the result between gatherings. The useful impacts were additionally investigated by a few examinations. At the point when utilized as one part of general sedation, nitrous oxide empowers a decrease in the necessities for different specialists, which are normally more costly and could make opposite side impacts (Becker 2008). Besides, a follow-up study showed that nitrous oxide diminished the gamble of industrious torment after a medical procedure (Chan 2011). These results were not evaluated in our Cochrane survey however ought to be thought about in clinical practice.

Cerebral venous apoplexy can result from hyper coagulation, either hereditary or gained. Hyperhomocysteninemia was recently remembered to be connected with thrombophilia, albeit this is as yet dubious to this current day. As of late, there has been a striking flood in the sporting utilization of nitrous oxide, which might actually prompt hyperhomocysteinemia. We present an instance of a 19-year-old female who was determined to have cerebral venous apoplexy with intracerebral drain. Cerebral venous apoplexy is one of the reasons for stroke in youthful patients and can bring about ischemic stroke, hemorrhagic change, and intraparenchymal discharge. The main sources of cerebral venous apoplexy incorporate oral prophylactic pills containing estrogen and hypercoagulable states [1]. Hyperhomocysteinemia is an intriguing reason for cerebral venous apoplexy [1]. Nonetheless, a few investigations have shown that hyperhomocysteinemia doesn't expand the gamble of venous apoplexy in the wake of adapting to bewildering factors [2-4]. Cobalamin inadequacy can prompt hyperhomocysteinemia [5]. Nitrous oxide, otherwise called snickering gas, has seen an expansion in sporting use lately. It can slow down cobalamin capability and cause hyperhomocysteinemia because of cobalamin lack [6]. Here, we report an instance of a lady with cerebral venous apoplexy with both cobalamin inadequacy and critical hyperhomocysteinemia coming about because of nitrous oxide misuse.

Case show

A 19-year-old female introduced to the emergency clinic with a three-day history of discombobulating. She had no huge clinical history except for revealed sporting utilization of nitrous oxide at a dose of 320 grams each day for quite a long time, and at a higher dose of 2,880 grams each day for one month before confirmation, without utilizing some other sporting medications. She denied utilizing oral prophylactic pills. She denied smoking and drinking liquor. She isn't a veggie lover and had a typical craving. There were no anomalies on the neurologic assessment. Beginning examinations uncovered gentle normocytic frailty (hemoglobin 10.5 g/dL, mean corpuscular volume (MCV) 91.6 fL, red cell dissemination width (RDW) 13.5%, WBC 6,780/μL, and platelet 177,000/μL). Following four hours of hospitalization, she fostered a summed up clonic tonic seizure, and diazepam and levetiracetam were directed alongside an endotracheal tube because of a trance (E1V1M1). Automated tomography (CT) of the cerebrum with contrast showed a few intraparenchymal hematomas (Figure (Figure1).1). The CT cerebral venography (CTV) uncovered broad intense intraluminal blood clot in the prevalent sagittal sinus, respective inward cerebral veins, the vein of Galen, straight sinus, sinus juncture, two-sided cross over sinuses, the passed on sigmoid sinus to the left upper interior jugular vein, and cortical veins at reciprocal high front parietal locales (Figures (Figures22- - 3).3). The determination of cerebral venous apoplexy bringing about intracerebral drain was made.

Intravenous unfractionated heparin (UFH) was directed and acclimated to keep up with restorative reach, with an actuated fractional thromboplastic time (aPTT) proportion (patient/control) of 1.5 to 2.5 for multi week, and afterward changed to subcutaneous bemiparin (low-atomic weight heparin (LMWH)).

As the patient was getting anticoagulant treatment, 1000 μg of vitamin B12 was subcutaneously infused day to day to keep draining from the intramuscular infusion. Seven days after every day subcutaneous vitamin B12 organization, serum vitamin B12 and homocysteine levels were estimated.

The patient was hospitalized for one month, during which time her awareness got back to business as usual and her engine power step by step improved to where she could perform fundamental exercises of everyday residing. All muscle engine power was grade V with the exception of left foot dorsiflexion, which was grade III. Because of the postponed recuperation of fringe shortcoming and deadness, a nerve conduction review (NCS) test was performed. The test uncovered predominantly axonal polyneuropathy with blended engine and tactile filaments. She was released with an arrangement for warfarin treatment for a long time according to incited venous thromboembolism. Vitamin B12 1000 μg was kept on being subcutaneously infused week by week for one month.

Conversation

We present an instance of broad cerebral venous apoplexy with intracerebral discharge in a youthful female with a background marked by nitrous oxide misuse. Examinations uncovered an essentially diminished serum cobalamin level and a raised serum homocysteine level. After cobalamin supplementation, the homocysteine level got back to business as usual. Other thrombophilia factors were not recognized, showing that hyperhomocysteinemia related with nitrous oxide misuse was the reasonable reason for cerebral venous apoplexy. She additionally had axonal polyneuropathy, which was reasonable brought about by cobalamin inadequacy.

Thrombophilia screening isn't suggested for patients with cerebral venous apoplexy by the European Foundation of

Nervous system science because of disputable proof in regards to its viability in decreasing mortality, working on practical results, or forestalling repetitive venous apoplexy. In any case, it is essential to ask about a background marked by estrogen-containing oral preventative pill use, which is emphatically connected with a 7.6-overlay expansion in the gamble of cerebral venous apoplexy [8]. The choice to direct thrombophilia screening ought to be individualized, as for our situation, where the patient had a background marked by nitrous oxide misuse that has been related with an expanded gamble of cerebral venous apoplexy. Thus, the serum level of homocysteine was estimated, uncovering hyperhomocysteinemia.

Homocysteine is a calculate the methionine cycle that is related with cobalamin, a typical regular coenzyme. The protein methionine synthase (MS) uses methylcobalamin and 5-methyltetrahydrofolate as cofactors to work with the change of homocysteine to methionine through methylation. At the point when cobalamin joins to MS, it is decreased to cob (I) alumni, the most receptive type of cobalamin, which moves a methyl bunch from 5-methyltetrahydrofolate, framing methylcobalamin and tetrahydrofolate. Methylcobalamin then, at that point, moves the methyl gathering to homocysteine, bringing about the creation of methionine. Nitrous oxide can change cob (I) alumni over completely to cob (II) alarming, which can't convey methyl gatherings. This forestalls the change of homocysteine to methionine, prompting hyperhomocysteinemia (Figure (Figure4)4) [6]. Nitrous oxide misuse has been accounted for to be related with thrombotic occasions, including ischemic stroke, intense coronary disorder, and venous thromboembolism. As far as anyone is concerned, there are six past case reports of thought nitrous oxide-actuated cerebral venous apoplexy in which pattern serum homocysteine and cobalamin levels were introduced (Table (Table2),2), and just two patients had cobalamin lack. In any case, it ought to be noticed that patients with serum cobalamin levels inside the ill-defined situation of 170-340 pg/mL could have cobalamin lack and ought to be tried for plasma methylmalonic corrosive or homocysteine levels, which are more delicate. The total blood count (CBC) could show no proof of megaloblastic sickliness or pancytopenia regardless of cobalamin lack, as was likewise seen for our situation. Our patient had blended engine and tangible filaments, which was because of cobalamin inadequacy. Because of fluctuating reports of measurement and span, it is trying to decipher the relationship be tween's the sum and length of nitrous oxide use and the seriousness of its belongings (Table (Table22).

EMONO is an equimolar combination of oxygen and nitrous oxide. In France, this is the main approved utilization of nitrous oxide for dental consideration. EMONO is enrolled on the French Public Office for the Security of Medications and Wellbeing Items rundown of medications with improved surveillance.1 ENOMO is shown in the absence of pain for excruciating demonstrations of brief length or during clinical help with grown-ups and kids, sedation in dental consideration in youngsters and delicate subjects, as well as in obstetrics. Its remedial worth was considered significant by the Haute Auto rite de santé — the French expert responsible for the guideline of the medical care framework. The ENOMO use has been approved in France beginning around 2001, however until 2009, it was saved for clinic use and the vehicles of the crisis clinical help administration. Beginning around 2009, an adjustment of approval for nitrous oxide-based claims to fame has approved their evacuation of the clinic save, which can now be given for proficient use in confidential clinical and dental practice. Today, it assumes a significant position in the French dental specialists' helpful weapons store for the dental consideration of resistant kids or with a handicap, restricting their collaboration. It permits us to keep those patients in a condition of cognizant sedation, most frequently working with care acknowledgment.

The EMONO as nitrous oxide, is a dismal and scentless gas. Absence of pain and tension are the two most looked for properties. For sure, in a cognizant patient, this medicine gives the decrease or disposal of torment and tension by acting straightforwardly on the focal sensory system with a lower impact on the respiratory system.2,3 More often than not, the clinical impact of EMONO inward breath is more unsurprising than other pharmacological means accessible in France, for example, oral cognizant sedation.4 The activity component of nitrous oxide contained in EMONO isn't yet completely comprehended, yet late examinations have somewhat clarified this system. The pain relieving impact is connected with the inhibitory impact of nitrous oxide on the N-methyl-D-aspartate receptors, which assume a significant part in the transmission of the nociceptive message and in hyperalgesia.5 Its invigorating impact on dopaminergic neurons has likewise been shown by the excitement of the emission of dopamine as well as norepinephrine, which are associated with the transduction of a portion of the impacts of nitrous oxide on the focal sensory system. Every one of the new outcomes have prompted the speculation that nitrous oxide actuates the arrival of endogenous narcotics in the periaqueductal dim matter. This is trailed by the enactment of narcotic receptors, γ-amino butyric corrosive sort A (GABAA) receptors, and noradrenergic pathways balancing nociceptive treatment at the spinal level. The speculation of the arrival of narcotic peptides is upheld by the center since morphine bad guys likewise somewhat estrange the pain relieving impacts of nitrous oxide.5 The anxiolytic impact includes initiation of the GABAA receptor, straightforwardly or in a roundabout way, through the benzodiazepine restricting site.8,9 The retention of nitrous oxide is speedy and happens through the alveoli. It is immediately discharged by the lungs. Lung assimilation and end of nitrous oxide are extremely quick because of its low dissolvability in the blood and tissues. This makes sense of the rate of the pain relieving and anxiolytic impacts appearance, as well as the speed of return to the underlying state after discontinuance of inhalation.10-14 As nitrous oxide is multiple times more dissolvable than nitrogen in the blood and dissemination hypoxia can occur.4 Accordingly, the nitrous oxide gas must be utilized in blend with oxygen, as on account of EMONO. It is extremely protected to use with no significant medical conditions distinguished when it is utilized in the suggested concentrations. Explicit examinations on EMONO have shown comparative results.

The pain relieving activity is by all accounts preferable known over the anxiolytic one. To be sure, clinical assessments connecting with this pharmacological substance are all the more habitually gone to its productivity in analgesia. Studies exploring the anxiolytic impact for the most part involved social scales for evaluating anxiolytics in kids during dental consideration, however as far as anyone is concerned, no review seeing this impact impartially has yet been accomplished in a youngster populace in dental consideration. A past report led at the Nantes Dental Consideration Place, entitled MEOPAeDent (imminent, uncontrolled, and homocentric), intended to portray the current, felt, and wanted impacts of EMONO during treatment emotionally by cross examination and perception of the child. Particularly we saw that just 62% of patients showed an anxiolytic impact, which showed up somewhat powerless for one of the two significant impacts that we could anticipate from EMONO. Additionally, absense of pain is likewise one of the known fundamental impacts of nitrous oxide. In this gathering of patients, absense of pain was felt by just 40% of patients. Be that as it may, anxiolysis and absense of pain were just connected with 33% of youngsters. Those outcomes, got from the kid's sentiments and correspondence, ought to be seen with alert, particularly since absense of pain and anxiolysis were hard to survey in this unique circumstance. In this way, the subjectivity of explanatory examinations is a predisposition that ought to prompt deciphering our outcomes with alert. As a matter of fact, it appeared to be essential to consider a more genuine evaluation of these significant impacts to explore the effectiveness of ENOMO. By and by, this study filled in as a reason for setting up this work and we will utilize it to make examinations.

Many examinations assessing the viability of nitrous oxide in medication or in dental consideration are based on a no inferiority plan. As a matter of fact, they looked at the consideration acknowledgment achievement rate between utilizing ENOMO or another sedative method or a placebo. They could likewise notice the patient's acknowledgment of this sort of sedation with negligible unfriendly effects. Moreover, social or potentially nervousness assessment scales are much of the time tracked down in examinations. The two most often found to survey the adequacy of EMONO stay the simple visual scale, whether for these pain relieving or anxiolytic properties and the Venham scale changed by Veerkamp for the anxiolytic effect. Thusly, current information from the distributed writing confirm an anxiolytic impact in youngsters utilizing EMONO. In any case, those appraisals stay abstract and, more often than not, contingent upon the agent as opposed to the patient. On the other hand, correspondence with the youthful patient is generally difficult and it very well may be challenging for them to offer their PCP a few clear responses to an oral survey about their inclination after this experience. Thus, those actions could be under or misjudged, which could change the evaluation of the impact.

We will look for through this work to concentrate on the anxiolytic impact of ENOMO, as would be considered normal in the youngster when it is utilized during dental consideration. This pilot study will endeavor to unbiasedly feature this by following changes in the HR of our young patients, which is perceived as a genuine pressure marker in kids and adults36-38 thus considered as intermediary proportions of nervousness in odontology. The EMONO influence on pressure will hence be acclimatized with its impact on the trepidation felt by the kid.

Materials and Strategies

Concentrate on Oversight

We directed an imminent uncontrolled monocentric pilot study to evaluate the EMONO anxiolytic impact in youngsters during dental consideration, called MOPEA. After accommodation, this study was permitted by the French Individual Assurance Board of trustees in January 2018. The information gathered during the test was dependent upon PC handling as per the prerequisites of the French Public Information Insurance Commission. It is additionally kept in clinical preliminaries (Novel Convention ID: RC17_0275).

Members

The example was chosen from youthful patients requiring EMONO sedation for dental consideration. Those rebellious or handicapped kids had restricted collaboration demonstrating cognizant sedation. To be incorporated, the patient likewise must be innocent towards EMONO and somewhere in the range of 3 and 15 years old. The consideration gave needed to include neighborhood sedation — consequently, we held patients requiring a dental separation or a pulpotomy.

The kid's cooperation in the convention was permitted subsequent to getting his/her educated assent and those regarding his/her legitimate agents. For the rest, the course of dental consideration actually stayed regular.

Systems

The review began in Walk 2018 and went on for 1 year at the Nantes Dental Consideration Place.

To notice our essential result, a HR screen was utilized when the kid was introduced to enlist his HR. This permits us to evaluate its varieties at various seasons of interest. It comprises of a straightforward PC with working programming and a scaled down sensor, for our situation, to be worn on the ear cartilage. Because of this gadget, a nonstop information recording was made. As a matter of fact, it permits us to notice changes in HR within the sight of outside upgrades, regardless of whether they are causing pressure. Toward the start of the meeting, the principal kid's uneasiness assessment by Venham scale adjusted by Veer Kamp was additionally made due.

Following the establishment, cognizant sedation with the inward breath of EMONO could start. Cognizant sedation is ordinarily accomplished following 5 minutes of inward breath. Thus, right now, another HR estimation permitted us to externalize the anxiolytic impact of EMONO on the kid. Then we began the actual treatment with neighborhood sedation. A last HR estimation was acknowledged during sedation, permitting us to feature in the event that EMONO changes the way of behaving of the youngster toward an unpleasant boost. Until the end of the meeting, we continued regularly for the rest of the treatment. At last, we eliminated the ear sensor from the HR screen and continued to the last youngster's nervousness assessment by the Venham scale altered by Veer Kamp toward the finish of the meeting.

Endpoints

The fundamental result of our review was to evaluate the EMONO anxiolytic impact in youngsters during dental treatment. Hence, our principal endpoint was the estimation of the subject's HR at three unmistakable minutes:

T0: Pulse (HR) during establishment — this action has been utilized as a control.

T1: Pulse (HR) following 5 minutes of EMONO inward breath — cognizant sedation, being by and large got following 5 minutes of inward breath; this estimation permits us to typify the anxiolytic impact of EMONO on the kid.

T2: Pulse (HR) during sedation — this estimation permits us to feature in the event that EMONO changes the way of behaving of the youngster confronting a distressing improvement — neighborhood sedation.

As an optional result, the examiner likewise surveys the kid's nervousness level toward the start and toward the finish of the meeting utilizing a Venham scale changed by Veer Kamp. This approved scale is the most generally utilized for the assessment of patient way of behaving during cognizant sedation care, with scores going from 0 to 5. " 0" portrays a casual kid, "1" an uncomfortable patient, "2" a strained kid, "3" a hesitant patient, "4" a kid inciting impedance, and "5" a beyond reach patient. The professional ought to rate the kid's tension in view of what he sees during the session.41

At last, as the third result, the information from the adjustment of HR will likewise be contrasted and the outcomes got utilizing this scale.

Measurable Examination

All the assessment boundaries were exposed to expressive examination. The quantitative variable assessment boundaries had been depicted utilizing position boundaries (mean or middle) and scattering (standard deviation, interquartile endlessly range). The subjective variable assessment boundaries were displayed as number and recurrence tables for every methodology.

An examination utilizing the chi-squared test was directed to feature contrasts between HR varieties at T0, T1, and T2. From there on unilabiate examinations were performed with the Wilcoxon test somewhere in the range of T0 and T1, T1 and T2, and T0 and T2. The circumstances for legitimacy were checked for the tests as a whole and the model.

An examination utilizing the Khi2 test was likewise led to feature contrasts in youngsters' degrees of stress between the start and the finish of the meeting. The information was registered utilizing Excel.

The consequences of the social scale show a slight improvement between the start and the finish of the meeting for the patients in our review. Scarcely any patients appear to be focused on toward the beginning, a vast majority of them have a score of 0 on the Venham scale changed by Veer Kamp. Be that as it may, those patients couldn't be treated in a customary way without cognizant sedation due to their tension. The great conduct the board related with cognizant sedation without commitment for the acknowledgment of the dental consideration (the patient realizes he can decline treatment after the initial 5 minutes of inward breath) at long last driven every one of the patients to acknowledge them. Thusly, it appears to be that the conduct scale isn't adequate to qualify the patients who will be challenging to make due.

Prud'homme et al. seen that as just 62% of patients introduced an anxiolytic impact, which was lower than we could expect for one of the EMONO major effects.28 By the by, these outcomes from the youngster's reactions are to be considered with alert, particularly on the grounds that anxiolysis stays a troublesome rule to survey in kids. In our review, a lessening in HR, which was the pointer that we decided to exhibit the anxiolytic impact, was viewed as in 80% of patients somewhere in the range of T0 and T1. Notwithstanding the pilot idea of the review, the pattern stays fascinating to show that, later on, this sort of more true assessment could be fascinating and ought to be summed up in examinations noticing EMONO impacts.

To be sure, the enrolled heartbeat rate varieties showed a genuinely huge diminishing in HR following 5 minutes of inward breath. In any case, the boost answerable for stress (sedation) is by all accounts apparent diversely as per the subject. A further lessening or support of the HR recurrence can be noticed. Toward the finish of the meeting, when the impacts of EMONO are scattered, there is a critical predominance of an expansion in HR, which might in fact get back to the underlying. This peculiarity could outline the finish of the anxiolytic impact acquired thanks to EMONO.

The achievement pace of dental consideration was 100 percent in our little example concentrate on patients not helping out customary consideration. This component, similar to the examinations recently did, shows that EMONO had an extraordinary spot in the restorative munitions stockpile of the pediatric dental specialist. In France, where midazolam isn't approved in that frame of mind of pediatric dentistry, it addresses the main choice for the dental specialist prior to proposing general sedation to numerous patients. Our review, accordingly, affirms ENOMO's essential interest. Notwithstanding, it very well may be viewed as that its utilization could be followed along by the estimation of HR variety during future examinations to more readily describe the uneasiness impact of EMONO.

This study permitted us to consider a better approach for expanding the assessment of youngsters' nervousness during dental consideration acknowledged with ENOMO. Previously, the acknowledgment of the specialized demonstration was the main variable saw to express the outcome of the remedial time. Then, at that point, the administrator could gauge the level of participation of the patient because of some assessment instrument, yet all the same that actually stayed emotional. To that end this option could be fascinating to have the option to follow patients' physiological capabilities in a more genuine manner.

Concentrate on Cutoff points

Two variables made the incorporations surprisingly troublesome. As a matter of some importance, our longing to complete the concentrate on youngsters gullible to

EMONO impacts extensively decreased the quantity of possibility for consideration. Countless kids found in the particular discussion for the no cooperative patient had previously encountered the EMONO impacts during their lifetime, in dental as well as in clinical consideration. In addition, a few youngsters wouldn't be remembered for the review due to ear-sensor wearing. This significantly slants the review and eliminates among the noncooperation kids, the individuals who are possibly the most restless.

The little example size decreases the extent of the ends that can be drawn from our review. This work, thusly, stays a pilot concentrate on that features specific patterns that need further examination. The absence of a benchmark group is likewise impeding. HR observing could be acted in kids having dental treatment without EMONO use to analyze the example of HR variety at T0, T1, and T2. The correlation would, in any case, be made between a collaborating youngster populace and a not coordinating one, which would restrict its advantage. We, thusly, didn't consider it important for this pilot study.

One more limit of the review is that the HR at T0 is taken during the establishment in the seat, which doesn't actually mirror the pattern level. The establishment on the dental specialist's seat, or even the basic appearance in the treatment room, can address pressure for the kid. Checking the HR a ways off from the meeting would be intriguing to defeat this issue and add an estimation before T0, however it would entangle the convention essentially.

At last, our patient populace shows critical heterogeneity concerning age. The portrayals of care and agony can subsequently differ altogether contingent upon the patient. The little size of the example further emphasizes the impacts of this heterogeneity on measurable investigation.

Viewpoints

In this review, we attempted to do an objective assessment of the anxiolytic impact of EMONO, which stays apparently, unpublished in France, where nitrous oxide is utilized here. The interest of this approach could be to propose later on deliberate checking of kids during dental consideration under cognizant sedation involving EMONO to have the option to rapidly typify its adequacy regarding the matter treated, in relationship with different devices accessible to the professional.

Additionally, Prud'homme et al. have shown that just 33% of youthful patients see all the while the anxiolytic and pain relieving impacts, which addresses not many patients regardless of the effectiveness of ENOMO permitting dental consideration. It very well may be fascinating to understand another preliminary surveying the absense of pain while enlisting the HR to assess the diminishing of pressure. Since this low rate could be owing to the way that kids were somewhat confounded after the dental consideration and had some trouble partner those two factors.

Equimolar combination of oxygen and nitrous oxide (EMONO), as we recalled during this work, possesses an especially significant spot in France. Proceeding with this pilot work on a bigger report or notwithstanding different investigations would be fascinating to approve the outcomes drawn from an example that tragically stays restricted.

Around four-fifths of Earth's environment is nitrogen, which was detached and perceived as a particular substance during early examinations of the air. Carl Wilhelm Scheele, a Swedish physicist, displayed in 1772 that air is a combination of two gases, one of which he called "fire air," since it upheld ignition, and the other "foul air," since it was left after the "fire air" had been spent. The "fire air" was, obviously, oxygen and the "foul air" nitrogen. At about a similar time, nitrogen likewise was perceived by a Scottish botanist, Daniel Rutherford (who was quick to distribute his discoveries), by the English physicist Henry Cavendish, and by the English pastor and researcher Joseph Priestley, who, with Scheele, is given credit for the disclosure of oxygen. Later work demonstrated the new gas to be a constituent of nitre, a typical name for potassium nitrate (KNO_3), and, as needs be, it was named nitrogen by the French physicist Jean-Antoine-Claude Chantal in 1790. Nitrogen previously was viewed as a compound component by Antoine-Laurent Lavoisier, whose clarification of the job of oxygen in burning in the long run toppled the phlogiston hypothesis, a wrong perspective on ignition that became famous in the mid eighteenth hundred years. The powerlessness of nitrogen to help life (Greek: zoe) drove

Lavoisier to name it azote, still what might be compared to nitrogen.

Event and appropriation

Among the components, nitrogen positions 6th in enormous overflow. The air of Earth comprises of 75.51 percent by weight (or 78.09 percent by volume) of nitrogen; this is the chief wellspring of nitrogen for business and industry. The climate additionally contains differing modest quantities of alkali and ammonium salts, as well as nitrogen oxides and nitric corrosive (the last substances being shaped in thunderstorms and in the gas powered motor). Free nitrogen is tracked down in numerous shooting stars; in gases of volcanoes, mines, and a few mineral springs; in the Sun; and in certain stars and nebulae.

Nitrogen likewise happens in mineral stores of nitre or saltpeter (potassium nitrate, KNO_3) and Chile saltpeter (sodium nitrate, $NaNO_3$), yet these stores exist in amounts that are entirely lacking for human requirements. One more material wealthy in nitrogen is guano, found in bat caves and in dry spots visited by birds. In mix, nitrogen is found in the downpour and soil as alkali and ammonium salts and in seawater as ammonium (NH_4^+), nitrite (NO_2^-), and nitrate (NO3−) particles. Nitrogen comprises on the normal around 16% by weight of the mind boggling natural mixtures known as proteins, present in every living life form. The normal overflow of nitrogen in Earth's hull is 0.3 part per 1,000. The enormous overflow — the assessed complete overflow known to man — is somewhere in the range of three and seven particles for every molecule of silicon, which is taken as the norm.

Essential nitrogen can be utilized as a dormant air for responses requiring the rejection of oxygen and dampness. In the fluid state, nitrogen has important cryogenic applications; with the exception of the gases hydrogen, methane, carbon monoxide, fluorine, and oxygen, essentially all synthetic substances have immaterial fume pressures at the limit of nitrogen and exist, accordingly, as translucent solids at that temperature.

In the synthetic business, nitrogen is utilized as a preventive of oxidation or other decay of an item, as an idle diluent of a receptive gas, as a transporter to eliminate intensity or synthetic compounds and as an inhibitor of fire or blasts. In the food business nitrogen gas is utilized to forestall waste through oxidation, shape, or bugs, and fluid nitrogen is utilized for freeze drying and for refrigeration frameworks. In the electrical business nitrogen is utilized to forestall oxidation and other substance responses, to compress link coats, and to protect engines. Nitrogen tracks down application in the metals business in welding, patching, and brazing, where it forestalls oxidation, carburization, and decarburization. As a nonreactive gas, nitrogen is utilized to make frothed — or extended — elastic, plastics, and elastomers, to act as a fuel gas for sprayers, and to compress fluid charges for response jets. In medication fast freezing with fluid nitrogen might be utilized to safeguard blood, bone marrow, tissue, microbes, and semen. Fluid nitrogen has likewise demonstrated valuable in cryogenic exploration.

Compounds

Albeit different applications are significant, by a long shot the best greater part of basic nitrogen is consumed in the production of nitrogen compounds. The triple connection between particles in the nitrogen atoms is areas of strength for so (kilocalories per mole, over two times that of sub-atomic hydrogen) that it is hard to make sub-atomic nitrogen go into different mixes.

The main business technique for fixing nitrogen (integrating essential nitrogen into compounds) is the Haber-Bosch process for blending smelling salts. This cycle was created during The Second Great War to decrease the reliance of Germany on Chilean nitrate. It includes the immediate union of alkali from its components.

Enormous amounts of nitrogen are utilized along with hydrogen to create smelling salts, NH3, a dismal gas with a sharp, bothering scent. The central business technique for orchestrating smelling salts is the Haber-Bosch process. Alkali is one of the two head nitrogen mixtures of business; it has various purposes in the assembling of other significant nitrogen compounds. An enormous piece of economically orchestrated smelling salts is changed over into nitric corrosive (HNO3) and nitrates, which are the salts and esters of nitric corrosive. Alkali is utilized in the smelling salts soft drink process (Solvay cycle) to deliver soft drink debris, Na2CO3. Smelling salts is likewise utilized in the readiness of hydrazine, N2H4, a lackluster fluid utilized as a rocket fuel and in numerous modern cycles.

Nitric corrosive is one better known business compound of nitrogen. A boring, exceptionally destructive fluid, it is tremendously utilized in the creation of manures, colors, medications, and explosives. Urea (CH4N2O) is the most widely recognized wellspring of nitrogen in composts. Ammonium nitrate (NH4NO3), a salt of alkali and nitric corrosive, is likewise utilized as a nitrogenous part of fake manures and, joined with fuel oil, as an unstable (ANFO).

With oxygen, nitrogen frames a few oxides, including nitrous oxide, N2O, in which nitrogen is in the +1 oxidation state; nitric oxide, NO, in which it is in the +2 state; and nitrogen dioxide, NO2, in which it is in the +4 state. A significant number of the nitrogen oxides are very unpredictable; they are prime wellsprings of contamination in the climate. Nitrous oxide, otherwise called giggling gas, is now and again utilized as a sedative; when breathed in it produces gentle mania. Nitric oxide responds quickly with oxygen to frame earthy colored nitrogen dioxide, a moderate in the production of nitric corrosive and a strong oxidizing specialist used in synthetic cycles and rocket fills.

Additionally of some significance are sure nitrides, solids framed by direct mix of metals with nitrogen, typically at raised temperatures. They incorporate solidifying specialists created when combination prepares are warmed in an air of smelling salts, a cycle called nit riding. Those of boron, titanium, zirconium, and tantalum have unique applications. One glasslike type of boron nitride (BN), for instance, is close to as hard as precious stone and less effectively oxidized as is helpful as a high-temperature rough.

Nitrogen structures a huge number of natural mixtures. The greater part of the referred to assortments might be viewed as gotten from smelling salts, hydrogen cyanide, cyanogen, and nitrous or nitric corrosive. The amines, amino acids, and amides, for instance, are gotten from or firmly connected with alkali. Dynamite and nitrocellulose are esters of nitric corrosive. Nitro compounds are gotten from the response (called nitration) between nitric corrosive and a natural compound. Nitrites are gotten from nitrous corrosive (HNO2). Nitroso compounds are acquired by the activity of nitrous corrosive on a natural compound. Purines and alkaloids are heterocyclic mixtures in which nitrogen replaces at least one carbon molecules.

Properties and response

Nitrogen is a vapid, scentless gas, which consolidates at −195.8 °C to a boring, portable fluid. Due to this high bond energy the actuation energy for response of sub-atomic nitrogen is normally extremely high, making nitrogen be somewhat latent to most reagents under customary circumstances. Besides, the high strength of the nitrogen particle contributes essentially to the thermodynamic flimsiness of numerous nitrogen compounds, in which the bonds, albeit sensibly solid, are definitely less so than those in sub-atomic nitrogen. Consequently, essential nitrogen seems to cover really the genuinely responsive nature of its singular iotas.

A somewhat late and startling disclosure is that nitrogen particles can act as ligands in complex coordination compounds. The perception that specific arrangements of ruthenium buildings can ingest climatic nitrogen has prompted trust that one day an easier and better technique for nitrogen obsession might be found.

A functioning type of nitrogen, probably containing free nitrogen molecules, can be made by entry of nitrogen gas at low strain through a high-pressure electrical release. The item sparkles with a yellow light and is significantly more receptive than customary sub-atomic nitrogen, joining with nuclear hydrogen and with sulfur, phosphorus, and different metals, and fit for breaking down nitric oxide, NO, to N_2 and O_2.

The five external shell electrons screen the atomic charge ineffectively, with the outcome that the successful atomic charge felt at the covalent range distance is somewhat high. In this manner nitrogen particles are moderately little in size and high in electronegativity, being halfway among carbon and oxygen in both of these properties. The electronic arrangement incorporates three half-filled external orbitals, which empower the iota to frame three covalent securities. The nitrogen particle ought to thusly be an exceptionally responsive animal types, joining with most different components to shape stable paired compounds, particularly when the other component is adequately disparate in electronegativity to give significant extremity to the securities. At the point when the other component is lower in electronegativity than nitrogen, the extremity gives halfway regrettable charge to the nitrogen particle, making its solitary pair electrons accessible for coordination. At the point when the other component is more electronegative, be that as it may, the subsequent fractional positive charge on nitrogen extraordinarily restricts the contributor properties of the particle. At the point when the bond extremity is low (inferable from the electronegativity of the other component being like that of nitrogen), numerous holding is incredibly preferred over single holding. On the off chance that difference of nuclear size forestalls such various holding, the single bond that structures is probably going to be moderately frail, and the compound is probably going to be temperamental concerning the free components. These holding qualities of nitrogen are recognizable in its overall science.

Insightful science

Frequently the level of nitrogen in gas blends not entirely settled by estimating the volume after any remaining parts have been consumed by compound reagents. Deterioration of nitrates by sulfuric corrosive within the sight of mercury frees nitric oxide, which can be estimated as a gas. Nitrogen is let out of natural mixtures when they are singed over copper oxide, and the free nitrogen can be estimated as a gas after other ignition items have been retained. The notable Kjeldahl technique for deciding the nitrogen content of natural mixtures includes absorption of the compound with concentrated sulfuric corrosive (alternatively containing mercury, or its oxide, and different salts, contingent upon the idea of the nitrogen compound). Along these lines, the nitrogen present is switched over completely to ammonium sulfate. Expansion of an abundance of sodium hydroxide delivers free alkali, which is gathered in standard corrosive; how much remaining corrosive, which has not responded with alkali, still up in the air by titration.

Natural and physiological importance

As may be normal considering the significance of the presence of nitrogen in living matter, most — while perhaps not all — natural nitrogen compounds are physiologically dynamic. Most living organic entities can't use nitrogen straightforwardly and should approach its mixtures. In this way the obsession of nitrogen is imperatively significant. In nature, two chief cycles of nitrogen obsession are known. One is the activity of electrical energy on the air, which separates nitrogen and oxygen particles, permitting the free molecules to shape nitric oxide, NO, and nitrogen dioxide, NO2. Nitrogen dioxide then responds with water as follows:

The nitric corrosive, HNO3, breaks down and comes to Earth with downpour as an extremely weaken arrangement. In time it turns out to be important for the consolidated nitrogen of the dirt, where it is killed, becoming nitrites and nitrates. The nitrogen content of developed soil is by and large enhanced and recharged misleadingly by composts containing nitrates and ammonium salts. Discharge and rot of creatures and plants return nitrogen mixtures to the dirt and air, and a few microorganisms in soil deteriorate nitrogen mixtures and return the component to the air.

Nitrogen itself, being idle, is harmless aside from when inhaled under tension, in which case it breaks down in the blood and other body liquids in higher than typical fixation. This in itself creates an opiate outcome, yet on the off chance that the tension is diminished too quickly, the overabundance nitrogen develops as air pockets of gas in different areas in the body. These can cause muscle and joint torment, swooning, halfway loss of motion, and even passing. These side effects are alluded to as "the curves," or decompression disorder. Jumpers, pilots, the people who work in profound caissons on whom the gaseous tension has been diminished excessively fast, and others compelled to inhale air under tension must in this way be very cautious that the strain is decreased to ordinary gradually following openness. This empowers the overabundance nitrogen to be delivered innocuously through the lungs without framing bubbles. A superior option is to substitute combinations of oxygen and helium for air. Helium is substantially less solvent in body liquids, and the risks are hence reduced.

Isotopes of nitrogen

Nitrogen exists as two stable isotopes, 14N (overflow 99.63 percent) and 15N (overflow 0.37 percent). These can be isolated by synthetic trade or by warm dispersion. Fake radioactive isotopes have masses of 10-13 and 16-24. The steadiest has a half-existence of something like 10 minutes. The main misleadingly incited atomic change was accounted for (1919) by an English physicist, Ernest Rutherford, who barraged nitrogen-14 with alpha particles to shape oxygen-17 cores and protons.

Somewhat intriguing, tantalum is similarly bountiful as uranium. It happens, with niobium, in the columbine-tantalite series (in which columbine [$FeNb_2O_6$] and tantalite [$FeTa_2O_6$] happen in profoundly factor proportions) and the pyrochlore-microlite series of minerals. Local tantalum metal with a few niobium and hints of manganese and gold happens sparingly in Russia in placers in the Ural Mountains and perhaps the Altai Mountains in Focal Asia. Rwanda is the world's biggest extractor of tantalum.

Tantalum is isolated from niobium intensifies by dissolvable extraction in a fluid cycle and is then decreased to metallic tantalum powder. The monstrous metal is created by powder metallurgy procedures. It can likewise be gotten by one or the other electrolysis of melded salts or decrease of flour buildings with an exceptionally responsive metal like sodium. The main purposes for tantalum are in electrolytic capacitors and consumption safe compound gear. Tantalum capacitors have the most noteworthy capacitance per unit volume of any capacitors and are utilized widely in scaled down electrical hardware. Different purposes remember getters and parts for electron cylinders, rectifiers, and prosthetic gadgets.

Tantalum is synthetically similar as niobium in light of the fact that both have comparable electronic designs and in light of the fact that the range of the tantalum particle is almost equivalent to that of niobium because of the lanthanides constriction. Tantalum is as a rule in the +5 oxidation state in its mixtures; lower oxidation states, particularly from +2 to +4, have been arranged. Tantalum compounds are moderately irrelevant economically, albeit the carbide Tack is utilized in solidified carbide apparatuses for machining hard metals. Virtually all normally happening tantalum is in one stable isotope, tantalum-181. In any case, a modest quantity, 0.012 percent, is tantalum-180, which has the surprising property of being tracked down in its energized state. The tantalum-180 energized state has a half-existence of more than 1.2×1015 years; the ground express (the most reduced energy state) has a half-existence of just 8.154 hours.

Helium

Helium (He), synthetic component, dormant gas of Gathering 18 (respectable gases) of the occasional table. The second lightest component (just hydrogen is lighter), helium is a vapid, scentless, and bland gas that becomes fluid at −268.9 °C (−452 °F). The bubbling and edges of freezing over of helium are lower than those of some other known substance. Helium is the main component that can't be cemented by adequate cooling at typical climatic tension; it is important to apply strain of 25 environments at a temperature of 1 K (−272 °C, or −458 °F) to change it over completely to its strong structure.

Helium was found in the vaporous climate encompassing the Sun by the French space expert Pierre Janssen, who recognized a dazzling yellow line in the range of the sun oriented chromosphere during an overshadowing in 1868; this line was at first accepted to address the component sodium. That very year the English stargazer Joseph Norman Locker noticed a yellow line in the sun based range that didn't compare to the realized D1 and D2 lines of sodium, thus he named it the D3 line. Locker reasoned that the D3 line was brought about by a component in the Sun that was obscure on the planet; he and the scientific expert Edward Frank land involved the Greek word for sun, Helios, in naming the component. The English scientific expert Sir William Ramsay found the presence of helium on Earth in 1895. Ramsay got an example of the uranium-bearing mineral cleveite, and, after exploring the gas delivered by warming the example, he found that an extraordinary dazzling yellow line in its range matched that of the D3 line saw in the range of the Sun; the new component of helium was in this way convincingly distinguished. In 1903 Ramsay and Frederick Soddy further resolved that helium is a result of the unconstrained deterioration of radioactive substances.

Overflow and isotopes

Helium comprises around 23% of the mass of the universe and is in this manner second in overflow to hydrogen in the universe. Helium is moved in stars, where it is orchestrated from hydrogen by atomic combination. In spite of the fact that helium happens in Earth's climate just to the degree of 1 section in 200,000 (0.0005 percent) and limited quantities happen in radioactive minerals, transient iron, and mineral springs, extraordinary volumes of helium are found as a part (up to 7.6 percent) in flammable gases in the US (particularly in Texas, New Mexico, Kansas, Oklahoma, Arizona, and Utah). More modest supplies have been found in Algeria, Australia, Poland, Qatar, and Russia. Common air holds back around 5 sections for every millions of helium, and Earth's covering is something like 8 sections for each billion.

The core of each and every helium molecule contains two protons, yet, just like with all components, isotopes of helium exist. The known isotopes of helium contain from one to six neutrons, so their mass numbers range from three to eight. Of these six isotopes, just those with mass quantities of three (helium-3, or 3He) and four (helium-4, or 4He) are steady; all the others are radioactive, rotting quickly into different substances. The helium that is available on Earth is definitely not an early stage part however has been created by radioactive rot. Alpha particles, shot out from the cores of heavier radioactive substances, are cores of the isotope helium-4. Helium doesn't gather in that frame of mind in the environment since Earth's gravity isn't adequate to forestall its slow departure into space. The hint of the isotope helium-3 on Earth is owing to the negative beta rot of the interesting hydrogen-3 isotope (tritium). Helium-4 is by a wide margin the most copious of the steady isotopes: helium-4 molecules dwarf those of helium-3 around 700,000:1 in barometrical helium and around 7,000,000:1 in specific helium-bearing minerals.

Made in the USA
Monee, IL
20 September 2023

43047708R00105